When Psychopharmacology Is Not Enough

About the Authors

Rebekka Lencer, MD, is a professor for Psychiatry and Psychotherapy at the University of Muenster, Germany. She has longstanding experience in treating patients with psychosis both with medication and psychotherapy. In her work with patients the aspect of taking the patient's perspective is fundamental. Besides clinical work she is engaged in research investigating cognitive impairments in this patient group.

Margret Harris, PhD, is a clinical research fellow in the Psychotic Disorders Program at the University of Illinois at Chicago. She has been specializing in the treatment of first episode psychosis patients using cognitive behavioral therapy. Collaborative relationships with patients and a strong emphasis on understanding patient histories and treatment expectations are fundamentals of her approach to therapy. Her research interests focus on cognitive dysfunction in psychosis patients early in the course of illness.

Peter Weiden, MD, is a professor of psychiatry at University of Illinois Medical Center. He has extensively written on the topic of adherence and relapse prevention for persons with schizophrenia. He has done some of the pivotal work on measurement and understanding of adherence problems for patients with schizophrenia. For his work on stigma, relapse prevention, and advocacy for the mentally ill, Dr. Weiden was named as a National Alliance for the Mentally Ill Exemplary Psychiatrist on three separate occasions. He is currently the principal investigator of an NIMH funded trial comparing a CBT approach with psychoeducation in patients with a recent diagnosis of schizophrenia.

Roland Vauth, MD, is the Executive Director of the Community Mental Health Centers of the University Hospital of Psychiatry in Basel, Switzerland. He is active as a behavior therapist, both in a supervisory and teaching role. Dr. Vauth's main areas of interest are schizophrenic, schizoaffective, and bipolar disorders, as well as sexual function disorders, eating disorders and adjustment disorders in chronically ill persons.

Rolf-Dieter Stieglitz, PhD, is Professor for Clinical Psychiatry at the University Hospital of Psychiatry Basel, Switzerland. He has extensive experience in the field of clinical psychology and psychiatric diagnosis and psychopathology with special interests in ADHS in adults and personality disorders, as well as the development of therapy programs for adults with ADHS and schizophrenic disorders. He is the author of over 400 articles and 25 books and psychological tests.

When Psychopharmacology Is Not Enough

Using Cognitive Behavioral Therapy Techniques for Persons With Persistent Psychosis

Rebekka Lencer[1,2,3]
Margret S. H. Harris[1]
Peter J. Weiden[1]
Rolf-Dieter Stieglitz[4]
Roland Vauth[4]

[1] Center for Cognitive Medicine, Department of Psychiatry, University of Illinois at Chicago, Chicago, IL, USA
[2] Psychiatry and Psychotherapy Clinic, University of Lübeck, Germany
[3] Psychiatry and Psychotherapy Clinic, University of Münster, Germany
[4] Psychiatric Outpatient Department, University Hospital of Psychiatry, Basel, Switzerland

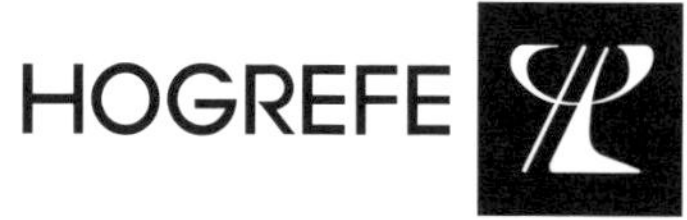

Library of Congress Cataloging in Publication

is available via the Library of Congress Marc Database under the
LC Control Number 2011921555

Library and Archives Canada Cataloguing in Publication

When psychopharmacology is not enough : using cognitive behavioral therapy techniques for persons with persistent psychosis / Rebekka Lencer ... [et al.].

Includes bibliographical references.
ISBN 978-0-88937-368-6

      1. Cognitive therapy. 2. Psychoses--Treatment.
I. Lencer, Rebekka

RC489.C63W44 2011   616.89'1425   C2011-900832-7

PUBLISHING OFFICES
USA: Hogrefe Publishing, 875 Massachusetts Avenue, 7th Floor, Cambridge, MA 02139
      Phone (866) 823-4726, Fax (617) 354-6875;
      E-mail customerservice@hogrefe-publishing.com
EUROPE: Hogrefe Publishing, Rohnsweg 25, 37085 Göttingen, Germany
      Phone +49 551 49609-0, Fax +49 551 49609-88,
      E-mail publishing@hogrefe.com

SALES & DISTRIBUTION
USA: Hogrefe Publishing, Customer Services Department,
      30 Amberwood Parkway, Ashland, OH 44805
      Phone (800) 228-3749, Fax (419) 281-6883,
      E-mail customerservice@hogrefe.com
EUROPE: Hogrefe Publishing, Rohnsweg 25, 37085 Göttingen, Germany
      Phone +49 551 49609-0, Fax +49 551 49609-88,
      E-mail publishing@hogrefe.com

OTHER OFFICES
CANADA: Hogrefe Publishing, 660 Eglinton Ave. East, Suite 119-514, Toronto,
      Ontario, M4G 2K2
SWITZERLAND: Hogrefe Publishing, Länggass-Strasse 76, CH-3000 Bern 9

Hogrefe Publishing
Incorporated and registered in the Commonwealth of Massachusetts, USA, and in Göttingen, Lower Saxony, Germany

Cover image:
"Umbrella Schizophrene" (1986), oil on canvas, 76 x 101 cm, by Bryan Charnley.
Reproduced by permission of Terence Charnley.

Printed and bound in the USA
ISBN 978-0-88937-368-6

Dedication

To our patients.
Thank you for sharing your experiences and for your dedication to the therapy process.

Cover Image

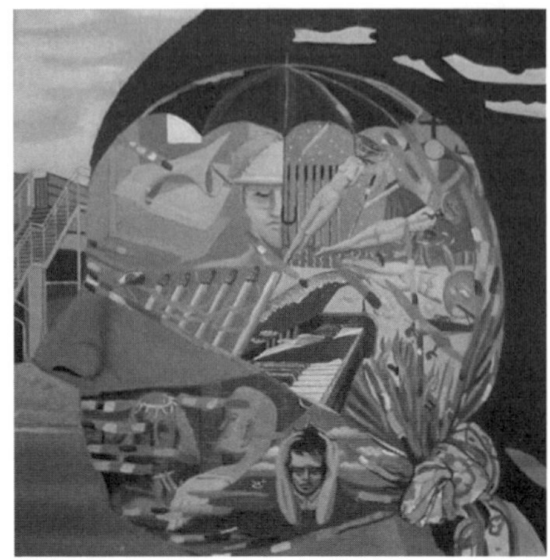

Bryan Charnley
Umbrella Schizophrene (1986)
Oil on canvas, 76 x 101 cm

The cover illustration is part of the work of artist Bryan Charnley, whose paintings vividly portray the effects of schizophrenia. The image of a head, blindfolded and gagged, with the mind exposed, stands as a powerful metaphor for schizophrenia. As many sufferers will testify, they are prisoners of their condition, which keeps them apart from society and bound within their own troubles. The sufferer is without a voice, and what he sees is disturbingly affected by his own mind. This experience is very difficult to communicate; the emotional and conceptual upheavals are invisible to the outside observer. In Umbrella Schizophrene, the ocean liner, waves, and piano keys stand as images for music, and more specifically, the ocean liner is a metaphor for the oceanic experience of music in which Bryan found great solace. Love and desire are represented by women as nails being driven into the center of the mind and then spinning downwards as though on a wheel. In an open field, a child's rocking horse stands abandoned.

Bryan Charnley was a gifted painter who intended his work to show the common humanity of the sufferer and how an artist can transform the most negative situations into the basis for creative inspiration. He was born on September 20, 1949, in Stockton-on-Tees, England. At the age of 17, he suffered from a first nervous breakdown that represented the beginning of his struggles with symptoms that would ultimately be diagnosed as schizophrenia. Although his formal art education was disrupted by his condition and periods of hospitalization and treatment, Bryan started painting and soon began to address his inner life, dreams, and mental states, particularly the nature of schizophrenia, in his work. The little recognition he received, however, was outweighed by the day-to-day problems of his illness and the heavy medication he was prescribed to counter these difficulties. In July 1991, Bryan Charnley committed suicide.

To learn more about Bryan Charnley's work and life, please visit the artist's website at http://www.bryancharnley.info/

Acknowledgments

Rebekka Lencer cordially thanks and is grateful to Fritz Hohagen for his encouragement to consider CBT a useful strategy for patients suffering from psychosis, and to Volker Arolt for sustained mentorship over nearly two decades in searching for the mechanisms of psychosis and new treatment approaches. Rebekka Lencer is also grateful to the German Alexander von Humboldt Foundation that made her cooperation with her colleagues from Chicago possible.

Margret Harris and Peter Weiden are deeply grateful to their United Kingdom CBT colleagues Alison Brabban, David Kingdon, Sara Tai, and Douglas Turkington for their intellectual generosity, guidance, perseverance, and mentorship over the last decade. Margret Harris and Peter Weiden were also supported in part by NIMH R34 MH080978 Medication Adhe-rence in Schizophrenia: Development of a CBT-based Intervention, and Katherine M. Ganaway Fund.

Rebekka Lencer, Margret Harris, and Peter Weiden would like to thank John Sweeney, Director of the Center for Cognitive Medicine, for his support of the CBT for psychosis program at the University of Illinois at Chicago.

Rolf-Dieter Stieglitz would like to thank Renate Gebhardt (Berlin, Germany) for waking his interest in patients with schizophrenia and for teaching him the first steps of CBT for psychosis.

Roland Vauth cordially thanks Prof. Hermann Rüpell (University of Cologne, Germany) for supporting his first steps into the field of research, and his parents for stimulating his curiosity. Roland Vauth is also grateful to the German Federal Ministry of Education and Research and the Swiss National Science Foundation for supporting important studies on this and related topics in schizophrenia.

Table of Contents

Preface to the American Edition (2010)

While the 1990s represented the "Decade of the Brain," its zeitgeist was captured in the primary reliance on psychopharmacology as the treatment for psychotic disorders. Until just recently in the United States, medications have been considered the only possible treatment option for persistent symptoms of schizophrenia. During the last 5 years, cognitive behavioral therapy (CBT) for psychosis has rapidly become accepted as an alternate treatment approach for patients with schizophrenia (when added to antipsychotic medication). A primary goal of CBT is to support patients in achieving their personal goals by taking their perspective. Consequently, this approach is more focused on symptoms rather than diagnoses and may help patients accept necessary treatment without risking a worsening of affective or suicidal symptoms. There is an entire new set of questions and challenges regarding how to integrate CBT and medication treatment, and how to choose between them, regardless of the practical reality that choosing between pharmacologic and psychosocial treatment options often depends on the availability of mental health clinicians trained in the psychosocial intervention.

A major contribution of the CBT approach to the treatment of psychosis to finally have an evidence-based nonpharmacological alternative for persistent symptoms of schizophrenia. In recent times in the US, the focus of attempts to address treatment-resistant symptoms has been almost exclusively on pharmacologic options. While there have been many pharmacologic advances over the past 20 years, the limitations of current pharmacologic approaches are also better understood. All of the authors of this present work believe that antipsychotic medications are overall needed for the treatment of psychotic disorders, and that once a diagnosis of schizophrenia is established, the advantages of ongoing antipsychotic medications almost always outweigh the disadvantages. However, as the title of this book suggests, medications are not enough. Persons with schizophrenia often continue to have disabling and distressing symptoms even while taking antipsychotic medications. In their efforts to emphasize the benefits, clinicians often do not fully appreciate the level of distress or discomfort that is connected with having to take these kinds of medications regularly and over many years. Bryan Charnley, the gifted artist whose painting is on the cover of this book, has also written about the suffering and havoc caused by his symptoms, and about the debilitating nature of the side effects of his prescribed medications (see http://www.bryancharnley.info/index.asp). From his perspective, there was no way out of the dilemma of oppressing symptoms and the feeling of dependency on antipsychotic medication. He committed suicide in 1991. At that time, CBT techniques, which are intended to help patients and therapists to find collaborative ways for more effective coping with the challenges of living with psychosis, were far from being therapeutic options. Almost 50 years after Aaron Beck described a first case of treating psychosis with CBT and nearly 20 years after Bryan Charnley's tragic death, more and more clinicians now consider CBT a valuable treatment for helping their patients.

The techniques introduced in this book will provide clinicians with a set of tools to first gain an adequate understanding of their patients' difficulties and struggles related to living with schizophrenia and having to adhere to a long-term medication regimen. Second, the book will lead clinicians to collaboratively work with their patients on facing these challenges and attempting new and often very creative ways of moving towards a more fulfilling and enjoyable life. In our experience, this approach has positive effects for the clinician as well, because clinicians feel more connected to their patients, and benefit from having more than one treatment approach at their disposal.

The previous version of our book was published in Germany in 2006 and was meant to be an introduction to CBT for German clinicians. Some of its contents have been reproduced in our book (Chapters 3 through 6), but we have taken the opportunity of this current edition to add new material that we believe might be of particular interest to our readers. Namely, a large section of this edition focuses on the integration of CBT and medication management for patients who might continuously experience distressing symptoms such as persistent delusions despite regular adherence to a medication regimen and patients who may choose not to take any medications. We have also expanded the appendices and strategy card selection from the German 2006 edition, to provide readers with assessment tools and session worksheets on medication adherence, for easy use in clinical practice. Although CBT techniques are useful for other psychotic conditions, in this book, we will focus on patients who are diagnosed within the schizophrenia spectrum disorders. The intended readership for this book includes not only physicians and psychologists, but also other mental health care providers such as social workers and nurses working with this patient group. Our hope is to encourage our readers to consider the CBT techniques introduced here as a useful tool for building closer and more trusting, but also empowering and productive relationships with their patients that will help instill hope, self-confidence, and a positive outlook.

Chicago, IL, USA and Münster, Germany, Fall 2010   Rebekka Lencer
Margret S. H. Harris
Peter J. Weiden

Preface to the German Edition (2006)

It is not only to Watzlawick (1989) that we owe the important insight that the ways in which we define problems in a clinical context often hinder their solutions. It is also our daily clinical experience that shows that it is often a different perspective, a different definition or view of a clinical problem that allows us to start working at a solution. This also applies to how we currently conceptualize hallucinations and delusional symptoms. The ICD-10 and DSM-IV merely provide a formal classification. These diagnostic systems are without a doubt a breakthrough for nosologic and differential-diagnostically clear classification according to uniform criteria. Also, the system for a psychopathological report introduced by the Association for Methodology and Documentation in Psychiatry (AMDP) has significantly contributed to a standardization of language in psychiatry and psychotherapy. Consequently, we can exchange information more efficiently and also weigh the results of clinical research based on a uniform diagnostic foundation.

However, this has led to a limited willingness in clinical practice to devote oneself to patients' subjectively experienced aspects of their symptoms – in our context, voice hearing and delusional fears. This may be irrelevant for a diagnostic classification or even for differential decision making in respect to psychopharmacologic therapies. However, it is inadequate when searching for a psychotherapeutic approach to chronic illness and to persistent symptom presentation in spite of neuroleptic treatment. Research by McCabe, Heath, Burns, and Priebe (2002), investigating routine psychiatric outpatient visits, clarified the following: During the currently typical 15-minute consultation practice session, the patient's subjective content of experiencing voices is as inconsequential as the subjective content of patient models explaining their changes in perception – what in clinical terminology is defined as a delusion. That stands in direct contrast to research findings that clearly show that a distinct focus on the patient in session will result in increased adherence, greater satisfaction with treatment, reduction in symptoms, and also reduction in emotional distress due to illness (Little et al., 2001).

But what is the cause for the current situation? The brief duration of appointments? No – we believe that this question requires a more complex answer. For a long time, psychotic experiences have been considered qualitatively different from the laws of everyday experiences to such an extent that a therapeutic approach based on patient experience seemed nonsensical. In addition, the helplessness and severity of disorganization of patients during acute phases of illness shape clinicians' views of the illness and its treatability. Acute phases of illness frequently require a paternalistic configuration of the doctor–patient relationship and to a great extent taking on responsibilities as a representative for the often much compromised patient. However, for long-term treatment approaches, this model of the doctor–patient relationship rather appears to be based on the stigma of the schizophrenia patient as a type of "big child." The lack of expectancy to win the patient as a partner in the treatment process who can contribute his or her own initiative and responsibility, leads to the dismissal of important chances for the formation of a therapeutic alliance. In addition, the noteworthy development of psychopharmacologic therapies over the past 10 years and the availability of second-generation antipsychotic medications with significantly better efficacy and side effect profiles have limited the focus on the subgroup of 25% to 30% of affected patients with schizophrenia and schizoaffective disorders who continuously and relatively persistently present with auditory hallucinations (voice hearing) and fixed delusional fears or systems. Further, over the past few years, research has been more likely to concentrate on early phases of illness – specifically, the early presentation of schizophrenic illness or first-episode schizophrenia. The underlying goal for this trend is to positively affect illness prognosis through early optimized treatment. All of this is appropriate and necessary but neglects the reality that persistent symptoms are not only a problem for individuals unwilling to engage in treatment but also still shape the lives of 25% to 30% of affected patients, despite progress in the understanding of neurobiological bases of the illness and further development of treatment options.

The contents of this book regarding voice hearing and delusions are exclusively limited to schizophrenia. Of course, patients with other psychiatric illnesses, such as mood disorders, also present with these symptoms. Of particular interest here are schizoaffective disorders, which are frequently combined with schizophrenia in research studies despite the fact that their nosologic status has not yet been completely determined. Our focus on schizophrenia is based on two factors: First, the greatest number of research studies exist for this group, and second, our own clinical experience is in this area. A number of the therapeutic interventions discussed will most likely also be applicable to or can be adapted to other disorders. However, efficacy has yet to be established.

Over the past 5–10 years, the trend away from conventional medical approaches to psychotherapeutic and psychological knowledge and towards an evidence-based view of disorders and their treatment has furthered modern psychology's analysis of the understanding of chronic voice hearing and persistent delusions as much as has the development of problem-specific methods in cognitive behavioral therapy. Although these techniques have been known for some time, they find embarrassingly little use in routine care. For the sake of our patients, these methods should be incorporated into the training curricula for behavioral therapies and psychotherapies, and future psychiatrists, clinical psychologists, and psychotherapists need to be educated in methods that apply to this field of practice. This book is meant to be a contribution to this goal.

Basel, Switzerland, Fall 2006

Roland Vauth
Rolf-Dieter Stieglitz

1 Review of Treatment Approaches for Psychosis

1.1 The Biomedical Model: Psychoeducation Directed Toward Medication Adherence

The concept of the patient as expert on his or her own illness can represent an important prerequisite for many components of successful treatment, such as shared decision making and cooperative work with treating clinicians, therapeutic goal setting, active cooperation in behavioral assignments or homework exercises, and medical decision making. As in the case of physicians treating most chronic diseases, clinicians treating patients with psychotic disorders should also aim to educate their clients about their illness, including symptom presentation and recognition, treatment options, and relapse prevention strategies. Psychoeducation is a systematic and structured behavioral intervention, providing didactic information about the illness and its treatment to patients, but also to family members. The approach also integrates emotional aspects into the treatment content in order to enable patients as well as family members to better cope with the illness (Bäuml & Pitschel-Walz, 2003). Thus, psychoeducation interventions represent a powerful strategy to inform patients of the risks and benefits associated with the self-management of their illness.

Psychoeducation is considered a widely adopted intervention for the treatment of schizophrenia (Rummel-Kluge, Pitschel-Walz, Bauml, & Kissling, 2006). Such interventions are offered in 72% of psychiatric hospitals in Germany, Austria, and Switzerland. In this subset of hospitals, only about 40% of inpatients with schizophrenia and 13% of their family members are reported to participate in psychoeducational programs. However, when considering all hospitals including those not providing psychoeducation, only about 21% of patients with schizophrenia and 2% of their family members receive such programs. *Underuse of interventions for families*, including psychoeducation, has not only been reported for Europe but also for the United States (Brent & Giuliano, 2007).

While psychoeducation for schizophrenia and other psychotic disorders is frequently used in clinical practice, it has generally not been sufficiently evaluated through empirical investigations. More recent reviews (Rummel-Kluge & Kissling, 2008) give us some evidence for psychoeducation as a powerful intervention for the treatment of psychotic disorders. Meta-analytic data have demonstrated efficacy for psychoeducation only when interventions included family members (Lincoln, Wilhelm, & Nestoriuc, 2007). That study showed medium effect sizes for relapse prevention and reduction in rehospitalization rates at posttreatment assessments when *both patients and family members received the intervention*, but only small effect sizes for the improvement of disorder-related and treatment-related knowledge in patients. In contrast, psychoeducation had no effect on symptom reduction, role functioning, or antipsychotic medication adherence. Effects for relapse prevention and decreased number of rehospitalizations remained significant for 12 months after treatment but failed significance tests for longer follow-up periods. Effects achieved for psychoeducation directed at patients alone were not significant.

Even a brief, eight-session psychoeducation program resulted in fewer hospitalizations and reduced lengths of inpatient treatment stays (Bäuml, Pitschel-Walz, Volz, Engel, & Kessling, 2007). Over the course of a 24-month follow-up, patients in the psychoeducation intervention group were hospitalized on average 1.5 times for 75 days compared to patients in the control group, who, on average, were hospitalized 2.9 times for 225 days. Aguglia, Pascolo-Fabrici, Bertossi, and Bassi (2007) replicated these findings in a randomized controlled study. Add-on psychoeducation programs for patients and families resulted in significantly fewer hospitalizations and days in the hospital after 1 year of treatment compared with a control group undergoing treatment as usual (TAU). In conclusion, efforts to integrate families into psychoeducational interventions appear to be essential for the success of the treatment. Whether psychoeducation directed solely at patients is also effective remains unclear, and further research is necessary.

Future treatment directions for the use of psychoeducation include joint groups of patients with different psychotic disorders – e.g., schizophrenia, psychotic bipolar disorder, and major depression with psychosis (Rummel-Kluge & Kissling, 2008). This intervention may not only be helpful for new, short-term psychoeducational approaches, but also for smaller psychiatric units with too few patients of the same diagnostic category to make separate treatment groups feasible. The content of session materials has also been updated to integrate issues relevant to providing culturally competent services, to address quality-of-life issues as well as gender-specific aspects of treatment. And most recently, peer-to-peer educational programs for patients and also for family members have been developed.

Cognitive behavioral therapy (CBT) approaches for the treatment of persons with persisting voices or delusional ideas suggest the development of a *working model* of illness in collaboration with the patient. This working model is developed through the negotiation between the therapist and the patient and their different perspectives. Traditional psychoeducation approaches, however,

frequently use the *vulnerability–stress model* of illness development to suggest that antipsychotic medications and their effects on biological causes of illness play a major role in symptom control and relapse prevention. This model has also been considered by some as helpful in reducing feelings of guilt and failure in patients when emphasizing the biological aspects of predisposition to illness expression. Additionally, by teaching patients about the importance of reduced stress for optimal symptom management, they learn that relapses are generally not an all-or-nothing phenomenon and that individual early warning signs usually precede acute episodes. When aware of their individual triggers, patients alone or with the help of family may thus more readily take charge of learning relapse prevention strategies and more easily engage in preparing crisis plans.

Yet, *nonadherence to medication regimens remains a large problem* throughout the course of treatment for patients with psychotic disorders, and no one existing treatment model, including psychoeducation, has been successful in significantly improving treatment adherence over extended periods of time. To improve adherence effectively, we have to think beyond the vulnerability–stress model and become familiar with patients' attitudes that may support or undermine the use of antipsychotic medication or other treatments for their psychotic illness. Only if we know these supporting or undermining attitudes will we be able to challenge them, using cognitive techniques (e.g., restructuring or inducing cognitive dissonance between goal attainment and nonadherence) or using motivational interviewing techniques (DiClemente, Bellino, & Neavins, 1999) to gently encourage changes in patients' adherence behaviors. Here, deficits in insight are addressed as anticipatory anxiety regulating behavior. For example, a motivational conflict may exist between the identity threat of being mentally ill and internally or externally stigmatized (Kleim, Vauth, Stieglitz, Corrigan, & Hayward, 2007; Vauth, Kleim, Wirtz, & Corrigan, 2007) and the anticipation of pharmacologic side effects. This may result in the conflict of objecting to medications on the one hand and desiring to avoid future relapses and their negative consequences (rehospitalization, loss of job and friends, etc.) on the other. Finally, *exploring the learning histories of patients' experiences* with their illness and how they have previously been engaged or disengaged in treatment is essential for adherence building in persons with schizophrenia. Only through the assessment of adjustment patterns to illness and attitudes toward medication adherence can adherence-improving strategies have a powerful and long-lasting impact.

Nonadherence to medication regimens remains a large problem

Exploring the learning histories of patients' experiences

1.2 Family Therapy

For many years, the effects of *family interaction patterns* have been regarded as *potentially significant triggers* for the onset of schizophrenia and also as modifying factors for the course of the illness, rather than being its primary cause. Above all, an important role is attributed to the concept of *expressed emotion,* which has been identified as a predictor for relapse in multiple studies (Butzlaff & Hooley, 1998). *Expressed emotion* refers to the communication of hostility, critical thoughts, or emotional overinvolvement by family members to the patient, resulting in increased stress and vulnerability to relapse. The focus of the family therapeutic approach is to foster change in the patient's social environment by providing psychoeducation to family members and correcting any false beliefs about the illness. This in turn can help in effectively adjusting attitudes toward the patient and the illness, and thus achieving a reduction in stress levels and an increase in coping ability for the whole family.

Family interaction patterns as potentially significant triggers

Expressed emotion

Behavioral therapy-oriented approaches used for family interventions have been developed by several working groups, the best known being that of Leff, Falloon, and Tarrier (review in Hahlweg & Wiedemann, 2002). In spite of differences across these individual approaches – e.g., with respect to setting

Table 1. Main psychotherapeutic elements of family management (Falloon, Boyd, & McGill, 1984)
• Psychoeducation
• Communication training
• Problem-solving training

(clinic versus home) or duration (6 to 24 sessions per year) – certain elements are common to all of these interventions, both with respect to the formal nature of the therapies and also in terms of basic content. All of these programs are characterized by a *very clear structure and highly organized session content.* The focus is on the "here and now" as well as *positive aspects and strengths of the family system,* and emphasizes the ability of families to bring about change. Session content includes three main components (see Table 1). Families receive psychoeducation with the goal of providing them with information and increasing their knowledge about schizophrenia. Further, communication and problem solving training aim to bring about an improvement in competencies and the personal responsibilities of all family members, and subsequently an improvement in everyone's quality of life. Ultimately, the aim is to facilitate relapse prevention goals and thus reduce relapse rates and number of rehospitalizations overall.

The theoretical background to the family management approach is based on the assumption that a recurrence of psychotic symptoms is likely to happen when tension and stress in the family environment exceed the patient's vulnerability threshold. Factors are assumed to be poor communication about problems within the family and ineffective problem solving strategies. By improving both communication skills and the ability to solve problems of all family members, the overall risk for relapse is expected to decrease. Additional strategies addressing specific problems such as anxiety, obsessive-compulsive symptoms, delusions, and hallucinations can be taught as needed.

To illustrate an example, the *family management approach* according to Falloon, Boyd, and McGill, (1984) is explained here in more detail. The first step of the intervention is a detailed behavior analysis of the family situation, including an assessment of strengths and weaknesses of the family as a problem solving unit, a description of relationships between the individual goals and problems of each family member, and observation of the family during the discussion of a problem. The actual treatment period consists of an information phase, communication training, and problem solving training. During the information or *psychoeducation* phase, families are provided with detailed information about the illness, including symptoms of psychosis, common causes, the frequency and course of the illness, options for medical treatment, and early warning signs for relapse. *Communication training* aims to teach basic techniques to improve the family's interactions, such as expression of positive or negative feelings and active listening. The subsequent *problem solving training* provides a multilevel, structured procedure for the solving of problems within the family, including collecting and discussing potential solutions, choosing the best solution, and implementing it. The significance of both training units and their interactions are shown in Figure 1.

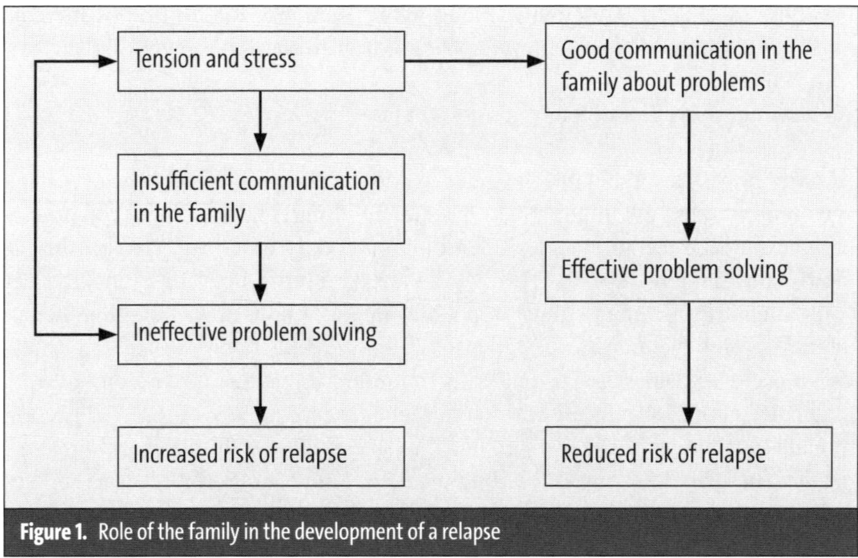

Figure 1. Role of the family in the development of a relapse

Evidence for family interventions has been well established over the past 30 years. With regard to efficacy, a number of reviews and meta-analyses (Hahlweg & Wiedmann, 1999; Solomon, 2000) have concluded that the use of behavioral therapy-oriented *family interventions can achieve a reduction in relapse* for at least 1 year. Falkai et al. (2006) point out that family therapy furthermore *encourages compliance with medication and may improve general social impairment and the levels of expressed emotion in the family.* Therefore several guidelines recommend family interventions in the treatment of schizophrenia, beginning either during the acute phase of illness, including in inpatient settings, or at a later time. For example according to the UK National Institute for Health and Clinical Excellence (NICE), an independent organization providing national guidelines for the treatment of diseases (National Institute for Health and Clinical Excellence (NICE), 2009), family interventions should be offered to all individuals who live with, or are in close contact with, a patient suffering from schizophrenia.

Family interventions can achieve a reduction in relapse

1.3 Personal Therapy: An Individualized Stepwise Treatment Approach

Hogarty's personal therapy (PT) (Hogarty, 2002; Hogarty et al., 1995) is a well-validated, disorder-specific therapy for schizophrenia that integrates a variety of efficacious psychotherapeutic principles, and can be tailored to different types of patients in relation to their symptomatology and level of impairment. The efficacy of PT for relapse prevention and adjustment to illness was evaluated in two 3-year trials, one for persons with schizophrenia living with their families and a second for those living alone. Results suggest improvements over time for patients receiving PT (Hogarty, 2002; Hogarty et al., 1995).

PT addresses three main aspects (Hogarty, 2002):

- disorder-relevant practice principles,

- the gradual staging of interventions by stepwise integration of increasingly sophisticated techniques according to patient's level of recovery, and
- affect dysregulation as a main treatment focus.

Hogarty postulates that a psychosocial approach designed to help patients manage their own distress might have a broader and longer lasting impact on relapse prevention than techniques designed to control only certain aspects of the patient's environment, e.g., the family. The regulation of affect represents the key component of this therapeutic approach. A range of both new strategies such as internal coping techniques, as well as more traditional strategies such as progressive muscle relaxation and social skills training, for managing stress and dysregulated affect are introduced in the treatment. Techniques are chosen to accommodate both the applicable phases of illness and also each individual patient's needs. The principles are offered as practical suggestions for a wide range of problems that may hinder stabilization, relapse prevention, and social recovery.

Stress management and affect regulation techniques

The primary goal of PT is to achieve and maintain clinical stability through a reduction in relapses by providing patients with *stress management and affect regulation techniques* that are linked to their stage of recovery from illness. Additional tools include the use of appropriate pharmacotherapy in combination with adaptive strategies appropriate for the management of potentially stressful relationships and life events that may act as triggers for illness exacerbation. To achieve these goals, PT is divided into three distinct phases as described by Hogarty et al. (1995): the basic phase, the intermediate phase, and the advanced phase. These phases were designed to accommodate a wide range of patients: from those recently discharged from inpatient settings, to those who have been living independently in the community for several years. The internal flexibility of this approach makes PT a true "disorder-relevant psychotherapy" for persons with a diagnosis of schizophrenia.

Components of the basic phase (Phase I) include:
- building a therapeutic alliance with the patient
- establishing a treatment plan
- basic elements of psychoeducation
- basic elements of social skills training.

Components of the intermediate phase (Phase II) include:
- maintenance of clinical stability
- personalized psychoeducation
- extended internal coping techniques
- introduction to relaxation techniques and additional social skills training.

Components of the advanced phase (Phase III) include:
- psychoeducation tailored to the patient's individual situation
- advanced internal coping techniques
- transition from solitary home activities to community reintegration.

Hogarty developed several criteria required for patients to meet for the transition from one phase to the next (Hogarty, 2002; Hogarty et al., 1995). Transition criteria for Phase I to Phase II include:

- successful maintenance of the prescribed antipsychotic medication dose
- a basic understanding of the illness
- sufficient sustained attention to permit participation in all components of Phase II – e.g., role-play scenes.

Criteria for the transition from Phase II to Phase III include
- gaining a basic understanding of the effects of stress on a vulnerable person
- completing homework assignments.

A process rating scale is used to assess whether or not the patient has met all criteria to move on to the next phase of treatment – e.g., items for the basic phase status involve (1) the patient takes medication as prescribed, (2) the patient knows one or more of his or her individual prodrome signs of psychotic relapse, and (3) the patient performs basic household tasks as expected.

In summary, PT can be characterized as an *evidence-based, phase-relevant, flexible individual psychotherapy for schizophrenia* (Fenton, 2000).

Evidence-based, phase-relevant, flexible individual psychotherapy for schizophrenia

1.4   Cognitive Remediation

Cognitive deficits in schizophrenia occur during early stages of the disease and most often remain throughout its course, mainly caused by prefrontal dysfunction in dopamine metabolism (Jann, 2004). Common deficits include reduced selective attention and maintenance of concentration over time, and deficits in verbal memory or working memory and learning (Ba, Zanello, Varnier, Koellner, & Merlo, 2008). Researchers have consistently found that 90% of persons with schizophrenia show meaningful deficits in at least one cognitive domain and that 75% show deficits in at least two domains of cognitive functioning (Bilder et al., 1995; Heaton et al., 1994; Palmer et al., 1997; Velligan & Miller, 1999). These deficits appear to persist even when the illness is in remission (Gold & Harvey, 1993; Sharma & Harvey, 2000).

Over the past 2 decades, a large number of studies have outlined the role of *cognitive impairment as a rate limiting factor* for psychosocial outcomes and response to psychosocial interventions in schizophrenia (Green, 1996; Green, Kern, Braff, & Mintz, 2000; Green & Nuechterlein, 1999). Therefore, focusing on these rate-limiting factors as therapeutic targets may improve psychosocial outcomes and expand rehabilitation readiness for people with schizophrenia (Green et al., 2000; Wiedl, 1999). Despite the fact that *second-generation antipsychotic medications* have been shown to be superior to first-generation antipsychotic medications in improving cognitive function (Keefe, Silva, Perkins, & Lieberman, 1999; Meltzer & McGurk, 1999), many cognitive impairments are not entirely normalized by treatment with these newer agents (Goldberg, Hyde, Kleinman, & Weinberger, 1993; Meltzer & McGurk, 1999; Weinberger, Aloia, Goldberg, & Berman, 1994). In spite of initial optimism about the improvement in medication treatment options (Ginsberg, Schooler, Buckley, Harvey, & Weiden, 2005; Harvey, 2006), more *recent studies failed to demonstrate persuasive efficacy of any drug treatments targeting cognitive deficits* in

Cognitive impairment as a rate limiting factor

Efficacy of any drug treatments targeting cognitive deficits are not demonstrated

schizophrenia, or they showed only moderate to low effect sizes, including for first-episode schizophrenia patients (Carpenter & Conley, 2007; Davidson et al., 2009; Keefe et al., 2004). Partial compliance may be the primary reason for the low efficacy of antipsychotic drug treatment, and the availability of long-acting injectable second-generation drugs such as olanzapine or risperidone may offer a novel opportunity to overcome nonadherence problems, as has been shown recently (Alam & Janicak, 2005; Burton, 2006; Houthoofd, Morrens, & Sabbe, 2008). However, it should be noted that even long-acting agents will not eliminate noncompliance. And further, medications alone are not sufficient for the improvement of cognitive function in patients with schizophrenia. The observed detrimental impact of cognitive impairment on day-to-day functioning and on the openness to psychotherapeutic and rehabilitative interventions has led to the development of cognitive rehabilitation techniques (Kern, Glynn, Horan, & Marder, 2009; Krabbendam & Aleman, 2003).

Cognitive remediation programs are designed to enable persons with schizophrenia to better cope with disabling aspects of cognitive dysfunction and subsequently increase their chances of achieving personal goals. In this role, cognitive remediation may be an important intervention prior to the beginning of CBT. The majority of cognitive remediation programs can be characterized as

(1) "cognition-enhancing" approaches, focusing on the improvement of cognitive impairments by repetitive laboratory-based exercises that are directly related to the cognitive domain being trained, or

(2) "compensatory" approaches, focusing on building compensatory cognitive strategies (Ben-Yishay & Diller, 1993).

Cognition-enhancing approaches based on the neuroplasticity model of brain development

More specifically, *cognition-enhancing approaches* aim at improving cognitive functioning through the stimulation of specific areas of impaired cognition. The approach is based on the *neuroplasticity model of brain development*, which assumes the brain's lifelong capacity for physical and functional change. Computer-based programs are most often used for this kind of training, although paper-and-pencil exercises can also be included. The training involves exercises designed to target a particular cognitive function such as selective attention. The trainer can modulate the difficulty of the task so that each individual is provided with challenging but realistic training tasks. The number and length of training sessions varies considerably across programs but typically involves two to five weekly 1-hour sessions over a period of up to 6 months. Results of outcome studies on computer-based programs for cognitive remediation in schizophrenia have generally been encouraging for improving targeted cognitive functions (Bell, Bryson, Greig, Corcoran, & Wexler, 2001; Kurtz, Moberg, Gur, & Gur, 2001; McGurk, Twamley, Sitzer, McHugo, & Mueser, 2007; Twamley, Jeste, & Bellack, 2003; Velligan, Kern, & Gold, 2006a). A recent meta-analysis of research on cognitive remediation (McGurk et al., 2007) reported a *medium effect size for improvement in cognition*, slightly lower levels for improvement in social functioning, and a small effect size for symptom improvement. Notably, effect sizes for studies in which cognitive remediation served as an adjunct to rehabilitation programs were higher than for studies using cognitive remediation techniques alone.

Although remediation programs have been shown to improve discrete cognitive functions in schizophrenia, there is a dearth of studies that include more real-world outcomes and longitudinal evaluation techniques (Krabbendam & Aleman, 2003). Only recently have researchers begun to focus on cognitive remediation as a method for improving response to therapy, e.g., social skills training (Spaulding et al., 1999) and in vocational rehabilitation settings as an adjunct therapy (Bell et al., 2001). In the latter study, patients were randomly assigned to one of two conditions: (1) work therapy alone for 15 to 20 hours per week or (2) work therapy combined with neurocognitive enhancement therapy for two to three sessions per week and up to 5 hours for 26 weeks. The computer-assisted cognitive exercises focused specifically on attention, memory, and executive functioning. Results show that patients receiving work therapy combined with neurocognitive enhancement therapy achieved *greater improvements in executive functioning, working memory, and affect recognition.* An investigation of cognitive training, integrated into vocational rehabilitation and focusing on strategy building and skill transfer to vocational functioning, demonstrated not only improvement in cognitive function but also showed higher rates of successful vocational and educational integration compared with vocational rehabilitation alone (Vauth et al., 2005). *Improvements in social functioning* through the use of cognitive remediation therapy has been reported by multiple investigators as detailed below (Eack, Hogarty, Greenwald, Hogarty, & Keshavan, 2007; Hogarty et al., 2004; Wykes et al., 2003).

Cognitive enhancement therapy (CET) (Eack et al., 2007; Hogarty et al., 2004), a 2-year therapy program, begins with 75 hours of computer-based cognitive exercises focusing on attention, memory, and problem-solving. The training progressively increases in complexity throughout the treatment. Following this first phase of treatment, 56 sessions of group-based training exercises are added for 1.5 hours per week. These group sessions focus on various aspects of social cognition, including communication, solving of real-life social conflicts, and appraisal of affect and social contexts. At 1-year follow-up, CET demonstrated marginal differences in cognitive style, social cognition, and social adjustment compared with supportive therapy alone. At *2-year follow-up, CET showed significant training effects* on neurocognition, social cognition, and social functioning relative to the comparison group.

Wykes et al. (2003) evaluated a *3-module cognitive remediation therapy (CRT)* addressing cognitive flexibility, working memory, and planning. CRT encompassed one-on-one instructions, with a strong emphasis on teaching methods that include procedural learning principles of errorless learning, targeted reinforcement, and mass practice using paper-and-pencil exercises. The same teaching methods were also used in the compensatory approaches described below. Training was conducted for 1 hour per day for 3–5 days per week, resulting in a total of 40 sessions. In contrast to an occupational training control group, CRT showed differential improvement on measures of executive functioning. Participants who met the criteria for reaching a specified threshold for improvement in cognitive flexibility also showed improvements in social functioning at a 3-month follow-up.

The *neuropsychological educational approach to remediation (NEAR)* (Hodge et al., 2008; Medalia, Revheim, & Herlands, 2009) is a hybrid approach that uses a top-down teaching approach emphasizing higher order strategy-based methods and the drill-and-practice types of exercises that focus on learning of more basic, elementary cognitive skills (bottom-up approach). The train-

Improvements in executive functioning, working memory, affect recognition, and social functioning

3-module cognitive remediation therapy

Neuropsychological educational approach

ing was conducted in two 1-hour sessions per week for 10–15 weeks. Results showed improvements in sustained attention, verbal memory, visual memory, and executive functioning, which persisted at 4-month follow-up. Partial support was also found for improvement in social and vocational functioning.

The computer-based cognitive remediation programs of Bell's and Mc-Gurk's groups (Bell, Tsang, Greig, & Bryson, 2009; McGurk, Mueser, & Pascaris, 2005) demonstrated *improvements in work functioning*. Patients receiving remediation therapy in addition to supportive employment showed a higher number of total hours worked and a greater percentage of employment compared with patients receiving supportive employment only. It is, however, difficult to attribute these gains to CRT alone because the programs included additional interventions such as cognitive assessment and job loss analysis, job search planning, remediative and compensatory cognitive skills training addressing on-the-job performance issues, and consultations with employment specialists and cognition specialists (McGurk et al., 2005).

In contrast to cognition-enhancing approaches, *compensatory approaches to cognitive remediation* "aim to bypass or 'compensate' for cognitive impairments by devising training methods to emphasize recruitment of relatively intact cognitive processes or by establishing supports or prosthetic devices in the environment to promote role functioning" (Kern et al., 2009, p. 353; Vauth, Dietl, Stieglitz, & Olbrich, 2000). As an example, 1–6 hours of "errorless learning" is directed toward eliminating errors during learning and response automation by bypassing deficits in the ability to self-correct. *Implicit but not explicit memory processes are stimulated.* Improvements have been demonstrated in entry-level job tasks, social problem solving abilities, and in different sheltered work settings (Kern, Green, Mintz, & Liberman, 2003; Kern, Liberman, Kopelowicz, Mintz, & Green, 2002).

A second example for compensatory approaches is presented by Velligan and colleagues (Draper, Stutes, Maples, & Velligan, 2009; Velligan et al., 2006c, 2009a,) in their work on cognitive adaptation training (CAT). CAT uses in-home environmental supports (e.g., alarms, signs, and checklists) and structures (e.g., reorganizing placement of belongings) to facilitate independent living in the home environment. This individualized intervention is based on an assessment of cognitive and behavioral functioning and focuses specifically on executive functioning. CAT was demonstrated to be effective in improving medication adherence and community functioning (Draper et al., 2009; Velligan et al., 2006c, 2009a).

Few studies have investigated *predictors of response to cognitive remediation interventions* in patients with schizophrenia. To date, predictor studies have used selected treatment outcome measures that were either part of the remediation intervention itself or closely linked to the intervention. Only a few studies investigated factors that predict generalization to measures of everyday life skills as an index for treatment-related improvement of role functioning in schizophrenia. A more recent study by Kurtz, Seltzer, Fujimoto, Shagan, & Wexler (2009) examined the factors that may predict changes on a performance-based measure for everyday life skills after 1 year of computer-assisted cognitive remediation offered as part of intensive outpatient rehabilitation treatment. Possible predictors of interest included in the analysis were four measures of neurocognitive function (crystallized verbal ability, auditory sustained attention and working memory, verbal learning and memory, and problem solving), two measures of psychopathology (total positive and negative symptom scores), and the process variables of treatment intensity and duration. Results revealed that auditory attention and working memory predicted changes in performance-based measures of everyday life skills, even when all other neurocognitive variables in the model and baseline life skill scores, symptoms, and treatment process variables were controlled for.

2 Moving Beyond a Biological Model

Current views characterizing schizophrenia as a brain disorder have dictated the use of a biomedical orientation for psychoeducation (Anderson, Hogarty, & Reiss, 1980). Biomedical models are widely accepted concepts for explaining and delivering treatment plans to patients, not only in the case of schizophrenia. They share the concept that a specific diagnosis, such as schizophrenia, has a final common pathway that causes significant abnormalities in central nervous system functioning. Consequently, *biomedical models tend to regard antipsychotic medication as the most important* and sometimes even the *single relevant possibility for treating brain dysfunction*. While biological approaches are very important, like all therapies they have limitations and shortcomings, and the potential complications that arise from communicating this disease concept to patients and caregivers may not be fully appreciated.

While we cannot say with absolute certainty what causes schizophrenia, *psychoeducation approaches require patients to acknowledge that they are ill* and suffer from a brain disorder. Overconfidence in theories of schizophrenia and psychosis has not gone out of style, although we cannot be absolutely sure that what we tell patients about their illness will be true 50 years from now. Current theories focus on the biological basis of the illness, and patients are often told that they cannot recover and that deterioration is common. Another "softer" version of this message is given when patients are told that untreated psychosis is neurotoxic to the brain, despite little evidence to substantiate this theory. This information is conveyed to patients with great enthusiasm, with the hope it will scare the person into taking antipsychotic medication. The point here is that it is not so much that treatment models are incompatible, but rigid and dogmatic statements that push patients into making forced choices when in fact they do not have to is more a reflection of our own stubbornness than it is the patients'.

It is widely accepted that many patients reject the label of schizophrenia and view their problems solely as being caused by stress, adverse life situations, or by the actions of others who wish them harm. In fact, one of the central problems to psychosocial interventions designed to improve treatment adherence in schizophrenia is the lack of insight and acknowledgment of existing difficulties related to the presence of an illness rather than due to external circumstances. This *lack of insight does not only present in patients,* but very frequently in family members and other caregivers as well. The use of the term *schizophrenia* or *psychosis* alone can create a significant barrier to engaging people to enter treatment.

An important reason for *patients* to reject a diagnosis of psychosis is the *attempt to maintain a functional image of the self* and to avoid an association with a highly stigmatized chronic mental illness. Patients who accept a diagnostic label of schizophrenia have been shown to have more depressive symptoms than those who do not (Rathod, Kingdon, Smith, & Turkington, 2005). Investigators in two European studies found that psychoeducation groups experienced more depressive symptoms (Carroll et al., 1999) and even suicidal ideation (Cunningham Owens et al., 2001) compared with CBT groups, and expressed caution about using psychoeducation because of these risks.

Another reason patients may reject a diagnosis of psychosis and subsequently treatment with antipsychotic medication is that *antipsychotic medications are not curative,* have limitations and adverse effects, and are not always as effective as clinicians would wish. Clinicians, however, may focus too much on the potential benefits of medications when discussing treatment plans with patients without realizing and/or considering what the patient's specific recovery goals are and, most importantly, how far the patient feels he or she still has to go to reach these goals, irrespective of medication adherence. Even with perfect adherence, taking antipsychotic medications does generally not lead to full remission, and *patients may be disappointed and frustrated by experiencing persistent symptoms or related deficits.*

One solution for overcoming the limitations of the biomedical approach is to *move beyond the "right" or "wrong" model of evaluating treatment approaches* and to develop a more integrative method that considers additional treatment techniques and their customized use in the therapeutic setting dependent on the situation of each individual patient. *CBT for psychosis tends to be more focused on symptoms than diagnosis* and may help the patient accept necessary treatment without at the same time risking a worsening of affective and suicidal symptoms (Sensky et al., 2000; Turkington, Kingdon, & Turner, 2002). CBT is perhaps more acceptable – or less demoralizing – for patients struggling with the personal meaning of what is happening to them.

A question that is frequently asked by clinicians new to CBT is whether or not patients with significant cognitive difficulties, such as memory deficits, attentional problems, and lack of cognitive flexibility, will be able to properly engage in therapy and follow especially the cognitive components of this treatment approach. Often clinicians voice the concern that CBT might be too demanding for such patients to truly benefit. However, clinical practice has shown this concern to be quite unfounded. The authors certainly believe that psychotic disorders such as schizophrenia are partially triggered by biological causes, such as hereditary predispositions. However, it is important for the CBT clinician not to overemphasize this fact during case conceptualization and treatment planning. To avoid inadvertent stigmatization of patients as individuals with permanent, biology-based deficits that cannot be helped, we would like to challenge clinicians to consciously maintain a neutral, stigma-free attitude and conceptualize patient difficulties in the context of anxiety and fear responses as well as intensified forms of normally occurring perceptual and thinking errors. This ensures that clinicians remain open for patients to bring up all and any difficulties when creating a treatment goal list and also avoids the exclusion of problems important to patients from the therapy process due to premature evaluation of these issues as "unfixable due to patient's inherent flaws" by the therapist. It has been our experience that patients not only highly appreciate an attitude of "nothing is off limits" but also tend to surprise

Antipsychotic medications are not curative

Move beyond the "right" or "wrong" model of evaluating treatment approaches

CBT for psychosis tends to be more focused on symptoms than diagnosis

therapists with their abilities to work through challenging issues, if given the chance.

Further, the use of *CBT techniques also offers unique opportunities for clinicians* compared to the biological model approach, particularly during the engagement phase of treatment for psychosis patients. While it is understood that psychotic disorders are partially due to biologically based causes, the CBT approach does not require a focus on this aspect and thus allows the clinician to avoid the potential harm that such a message might do to clinician–patient rapport. Instead, clinicians are able to truly engage in patient-centered practice by *focusing on the patient's experiences, worries and fears, and specific treatment goals* and collaboratively create a treatment plan that focuses on patient strengths and may incorporate antipsychotic medications as one of multiple tools available to the patient in his or her recovery. This active involvement of the patient and focus on self-empowerment conveys the message of truly individualized treatment and strong interest of the clinician in the patient's unique circumstances, rather than a generic-appearing response of only prescribing medications. In turn, clinicians feel more connected to their patients, see greater willingness to engage, and benefit from having more than one treatment approach at their disposal.

CBT can be used alongside most biological models of schizophrenia. It is perfectly acceptable for a psychiatric practitioner to believe in a biological/medical causation of schizophrenia and still embrace a cognitive behavioral model to use with patient care. Although a cognitive behavioral approach would not contradict a biological point of view in a patient whose personal explanation fits that model, it does not insist on it for patients who prefer other explanations. Therefore, CBT is not compatible with any kind of biomedically based intervention that requires using the diagnostic label "schizophrenia," forbids any exploration of a personal meaning (formulation) of psychotic symptoms, or precludes the possibility of meaningful recovery.

One of the potential benefits of taking a CBT approach over a more traditional "medical model" approach is that it may selectively engage some individuals into accepting treatment and antipsychotic medication. A psychotherapeutic intervention such as CBT, which focuses on the relationship and the person's own life situation in a way that normalizes his or her symptoms and predicament may *lead to a better therapeutic alliance* and ultimately better insight into the important role of medication in maintaining wellness.

The literature shows a strong relationship between the therapeutic alliance, medication compliance, and outcome for patients with schizophrenia. However, this association only holds when the patient is taking antipsychotic medication in the first place. What does this tell us? At the very least, it tells us that, while medications are important, they are often not enough on their own. Patients who have good relationships with their prescribing doctors are more likely to stay on medication, less likely to relapse, and generally will do better in other aspects of life (Frank & Gunderson, 1990).

Focusing on the patient's experiences, worries and fears, and specific treatment goals

CBT can be used alongside most biological models

Better therapeutic alliance

3 Evidence Supporting the Use of Cognitive Behavioral Therapy for Psychosis

Recent meta-analyses (Wykes, Steel, Everitt, & Tarrier, 2008; Zimmermann, Favrod, Trieu, & Pomini, 2005) underline the effectiveness of interventions for persistent voices and chronic delusions that are based on CBT strategies and that are offered to patients as adjuncts to antipsychotic treatment. In clinical practice, CBT strategies are recommended by the guidelines for the treatment and management of schizophrenia in primary and secondary care provided by NICE in the United Kingdom (NICE, 2009), by the treatment recommendations formulated by the Patient Outcome Research Team (Kreyenbuhl, Buchanan, Dickerson, & Dixon, 2010), and early practice guidelines for the treatment of patients with schizophrenia provided by the American Psychiatric Association Steering Committee (2004). With the goal of giving our readers an overview of the empirical evidence for the use of CBT for psychosis for patients with persistent delusions, we will address the following open questions:

- What exactly is the evidence for using cognitive behavioral interventions for persistent positive symptoms in schizophrenia?
- What are the results of the most recent randomized control trials and meta-analyses?
- What is the impact of these interventions on what specific therapeutic target?
- What are their limits?
- What are the shortcomings of the included studies?

The most recent meta-analysis (Wykes et al., 2008) is based on 34 randomized controlled trials and thus includes 20 more trials and 475 more participants than previous meta-analyses on cognitive behavioral interventions for psychosis (Zimmermann et al., 2005). Wykes et al. (2008) found an effect size of 0.40 (95% confidence interval: 0.25–0.55) for overall beneficial effects of CBT for psychosis. The level of efficacy and number of studies supporting efficacy differed depending on target symptoms. Thirty-two studies supported efficacy in the reduction of positive symptoms, and 23 studies reported reduction of negative symptoms. Furthermore, there were beneficial effects for functional outcome (15 studies), improvement in mood symptoms (13 studies), and reduction in social anxiety (2 studies), with effect sizes ranging from 0.35 to 0.44. Also, the studies that were included improved in quality (more rigorously controlled trials) and sample size over time. Most importantly, effect sizes depended on the strength of control conditions (e.g., what kind of treatment was defined as usual) and on the methodological rigor of the study. Rating of the methodological quality was assessed by the clinical trial assessment measure (CTAM). The CTAM includes criteria such as the strategy to control for selection bias in recruitment, sample size based on adequate power calculations, appropriate and clearly described random allocation to treatment condition, use of standardized assessment methods, collection of participants independently of treatment by assessors who are unaware of treatment allocation, control for nonspecific effects of treatment by including a placebo attention control condition in the study design (e.g., befriending), use of a treatment manual or protocol so that interventions can be independently replicated by other research groups, use of fidelity scales to measure adherence to the manual, and selection of adequate statistical methods in data analysis (e.g., intention-to-treat analyses in spite of last observation carried forward, etc.). Studies in which raters were aware of group allocation had inflated effect sizes between 50% and 100%. The authors concluded that missing blind assessment of outcome (no mask of treatment allocation) may overestimate the effect size of the treatment (Wykes et al., 2008).

Other studies investigating the treatment efficacy of CBT interventions for psychosis identified improvements in adherence to pharmacologic treatment regime (Kemp, Hayward, Applewhaite, Everitt, & David, 1996), improvements in overall level of insight, symptoms of psychosis, symptoms of depression (Turkington et al., 2002), and longer intervals to next hospitalization (Turkington et al., 2006a). This effect was maintained at a 24-month follow-up; however, vocational functioning did not improve (Malik, Kingdon, Pelton, Mehta, & Turkington, 2009). Additional studies demonstrated benefits of CBT interventions for the reduction of relapse frequency (Gumley et al., 2003), but in trials in which hospitalization was excluded as proxy for relapse, CBT seemed not to have an effect (Lynch, Laws, & McKenna, 2010).

There are several limitations to the currently available studies. Given the heterogeneity of interventions used across different research groups investigating the efficacy of CBT interventions for persistent positive symptoms of psychosis, the potential mechanisms of action that are effective in successful therapeutic interventions remain unclear. So-called dismantling strategies, which compare systematic variations of different subsets of treatment modules, are missing. Additionally, neurobiologically based analyses that are able to reveal functional changes in the brain that correlate with therapeutic response or nonresponse (e.g., functional magnetic resonance imaging (fMRI)) are not yet used for the evaluation of treatment methods.

However, some progress in these areas has been made. Morrison and Barratt (2010) applied the Delphi method (a systematic, interactive forecasting method) to identify those intrinsic components of CBT for psychosis deemed most important by a panel of 28 experts on CBT for psychosis. Following this approach, more than 80% of these clinical academics and highly trained trial therapists identified 77 items as essential to CTB for psychosis in three rounds of producing and rating statements that addressed issues such as case formulation, coping strategy enhancement, homework assignments, and identifying individual positive and personally relevant treatment goals.

A set of other studies identified predictors for the response to CBT for psychosis strategies, including a shorter duration of untreated psychosis, female sex (Drury, Birchwood, Cochrane, & Macmillan, 1996), a higher level of insight, a higher number of hospital admissions (Garety et al., 1997), and lower level of conviction in delusions (Brabban, Tai, & Turkington, 2009).

Few investigations exist to date that have attempted to identify neurobiological correlates of improvement of schizophrenia symptoms through the use of CBT for psychosis techniques. Premkumar et al. (2009) found that a reduction in positive symptoms of schizophrenia was associated with greater right cerebellum gray matter volume, a reduction in negative symptoms was associated with left precentral gyrus and right inferior parietal lobule gray matter volumes, and a reduction in general psychopathology was associated with greater right superior temporal gyrus, cuneus, and cerebellum gray matter volumes. The authors concluded that gray matter volumes of the frontal, temporal, parietal, and cerebellar areas, which are known to be involved in the coordination of mental activity, cognitive flexibility, and verbal learning and memory, are able to predict responsiveness to CBT in patients with psychosis. Also, stronger dorsolateral prefrontal cortex activity and connectivity with the cerebellum predicted greater responsiveness to CBT in schizophrenia patients (Kumari et al., 2009). Further, findings of an fMRI study (Kumari et al., 2010) showed changes in language processing, attention, insight, and self-awareness for schizophrenia patients after CBT for psychosis treatment.

In summary, while some existing studies show certain methodological flaws, strong evidence exists that CBT for psychosis is an effective treatment for persistent positive symptoms in schizophrenia. The majority of treated patients improved on several outcome domains after receiving this therapeutic intervention. Given the fact that 20% to 25% of patients who suffer from positive symptoms are only partial treatment responders, although they are adherent to optimal pharmacologic treatment, we should expand the delivery of CBT intervention programs for patients with persistent positive symptoms of schizophrenia, such as delusions, especially in outpatient treatment settings.

4 General Aspects of Treatment

4.1 Treatment Goals and Treatment Components

Although individual CBT approaches for the treatment of chronic positive symptoms may differ in terms of content and with regard to target symptoms and treatment strategies, they do show a number of important *similarities*:

Similarities in Cognitive Behavioral Approaches

- Emphasis on the significance of building a *strong therapeutic relationship* by providing acceptance and support as well as the collaborative approach to problems
- Development and *hierarchization of a problem list* with regard to symptoms and life goals

The first sessions in particular should serve to create a good and sustainable working relationship and to establish achievable and therefore motivating therapy goals. The *determination of roles* for the therapist and patient should have substantial significance in the initial phase of treatment, with the goal of establishing a partnership-based working relationship. The clinician fills the role of a helpful guide for the patient throughout the collaborative therapy process, rather than that of an expert making all treatment decisions alone.

Psychoeducation techniques, which are primarily based on the *normalizing approach* – e.g., the psychotic experience is conceptualized as "sensitivity illness" (Kingdon, 1998) – can help clarify the role of stress in light of any existing illness predisposition as well as insufficient protective factors while reducing stigma at the same time. In addition to the negotiation of therapy objectives, the goal of the initial treatment phase is to *foster a collaborative problem-understanding* by means of the development of a working model. This conceptualizes the patient's problems as a vicious cycle which includes specific triggers and perpetuating factors analogous to the cycle seen in panic disorders. The goal is to increase the possibilities of affecting and controlling symptoms for both the patient and his or her social supporters, thereby reducing stress effects. In addition, the normalizing strategy should decrease internally generated stigma and shame caused by psychotic symptoms such as voice hearing. This last aspect is essential for the patient's motivation regarding whether or not to engage in treatment.

Positive and negative symptoms will be addressed by means of *cognitive behavioral techniques*. Examples include Socratic questioning, cognitive restructuring, identification of alternative explanations, behavioral experiments, therapeutically led self-confrontation (exposition), and role plays. *Emotions resulting from persistent positive symptoms,* such as fear and depression, are the focus of treatment through strategies such as relaxation techniques, self-confrontation, the identification of evaluative processes, or the improvement of time structuring.

Table 2. Goals of cognitive therapy for delusions and voice hearing

• Fostering problem-understanding
• Reduction of negative effects of the symptoms on the concept of self
• Improvement of adaptation to symptoms:
  – role functioning
  – support during the resolution of age-appropriate developmental tasks
• Reduction of the risk for comorbidities such as
  – addiction
  – depression
  – social phobia
• Relapse prevention
• Teaching of coping strategies for managing chronic positive symptoms
Adapted from Rector & Beck (2002)

For *relapse prevention,* treatment goals include the better management of symptom triggers for which the patient shows increased vulnerability. This includes changing of dysfunctional "interpersonal scenarios" (Morrison, 1998), skills training, and the development and practice of a crisis plan (Herz et al., 2000). In addition, a stepwise plan for the management of setbacks will be developed.

Relapse prevention

The general treatment goals of cognitive therapy for delusions and voice hearing are summarized in Table 2.

The second goal after fostering an understanding of the problem is the *reduction of negative effects of the symptoms on the patient's self-image.* For example, deprecating voices or ongoing persecutory delusions can substantially decrease self-esteem. Techniques such as the "empty chair," imagination of counterarguments (e.g., How do you defend yourself against insults from a neighbor?), reality testing, and other cognitive strategies are used here.

Reduction of negative effects of the symptoms on the patient's self-image

Thirdly, the *adaptation to symptoms* should be improved in two ways: role functioning at home or in the work environment as well as age-appropriate resolution of developmental tasks (e.g., gaining independence from the parental home, relationships, and job training). The *negative effects of symptoms should be reduced* through teaching or improving appropriate coping strategies. Examples include the reduction of secondary addictions, of the development of depressive syndromes with increased suicide risk, and of social withdrawal. The elements of CBT designed to achieve these objectives are summarized in Table 3 and discussed in detail below.

Adaptation to symptoms

At the start of any therapy, individualized joint *therapeutic goals, or problem lists,* must be identified and formulated with the patient. The goal formulation must, however, fulfill specific criteria to be efficient. Target items on the problem list must have the following features: They must be

Joint therapeutic goals or problem lists

- *positive:* not simply "hear fewer voices", but also define how this type of life with fewer voices will be more attractive to the patient
- *achievable:* consider resources *and* obstacles appropriately
- *behavior based:* based on which behavior or which criteria does one recognize the achievement of the goal?
- formulated to be *subjectively attractive.*

Table 3. Elements of cognitive therapy for delusions and voice hearing
• Establish a strong therapeutic alliance: acceptance, support, collaborative approach to problems
• Develop and prioritize a problem list: symptoms, life goals
• Psychoeducation and normalizing symptoms: reduction of stigma, emphasis on the role of stress and biopsychosocial factors
• Develop a collaborative model with the patient: themes of the problem list, processing of "vicious cycles" (identify links between thoughts, feelings, and behavior)
• Focus on positive and negative symptoms using cognitive behavioral techniques such as Socratic questioning, cognitive restructuring, reality testing, identifying alternative explanations, behavioral experiments, eliciting self-beliefs, investigating fear/suspicion hierarchies, and use of imagery and role plays
• Focus on comorbid depression and anxiety using cognitive behavioral techniques such as relaxation exercises, creating weekly activity schedules and exposure exercises, focusing on misinterpretations, and testing and reframing beliefs related to anxiety and depression
• Relapse prevention: identifying high-risk situations, skills training, and crisis plan
• Establish stepwise action plan to deal with setbacks
Adapted from (Rector & Beck, 2002)

Notably, to be less burdened by the hearing of voices or by delusional fears alone is not in and of itself a sufficiently clear goal of therapy. For therapy planning, the question is always important: What does the patient wish to achieve in concrete terms by means of improved symptom control in his or her life? Proven strategies to foster collaborative work on a problem list and related therapy goals can be found in Table 4.

Table 4. Strategies to promote the collaborative development of a problem list and treatment plan
• Identification of situations which disturb or burden the patient, as a starting point to build support and motivation
• Practical assistance
• Therapist as guide through the therapeutic process
• Delay of the therapist's wish for agreement about the diagnosis
• Encouragement and conveying of hope

4.2 Planning of Treatment Sessions

The typical course of sessions generally includes six phases as outlined in Table 5.

Development of the goal symptoms

The *development of the goal symptoms* since the last session, e.g., invasiveness of aggressive voices, depressed state of mind, or anxiety regarding delusional fears, can be captured using self-observation protocols such as symp-

Table 5. Typical cognitive therapy session (25–50 min)

- *Progress Update*
  - Update on mood since last session (may complete brief mood ratings survey)
  - Medication adherence
  - Improvements
  - Use of help and services
- *Bridge to last session*
  - Summary of previous session's most important issues and conclusions
  - Set agenda for current session
- *Working through session agenda*, e.g.:
  - applying cognitive strategies targeting delusions
  - devising and carrying out behavioral experiment to test beliefs about voices
  - practicing coping strategies for managing unanticipated crises
- *Planning and agreeing on homework assignments* until next session
- *Summary and patient's feedback* on session
  - What can/will patient carry forward from this session?
  - What was helpful?
  - What remains unresolved?
- *Repeated overview* of steps until next session and clarification of connections to the overall treatment plan (benefits, goals, etc.)

Adapted from Rector & Beck (2002)

tom diaries. This is particularly useful for patients in order to develop a sense for which situations present an increased vulnerability to specific symptoms and which situations present as protective factors. Regular documentation of changes in goal symptoms can contribute significantly to patients' motivation (hope for success) because they maintain a record of their personal progress. During the *review* of the previous session, the therapist must test whether or not the patient has understood what was discussed and agreed upon with regard to the main themes of therapy.

Next, a *topic list for the current session* should be developed. In the case of patients who are cognitively or emotionally impaired, it might be necessary to reduce the session length to 20–35 minutes and to concentrate on a single core topic. Disturbance- and problem-specific techniques should be used, such as training of coping strategies aiming to better manage invasive voices, planning of behavioral experiments to examine delusional fears, and self confrontations under guidance by the therapist. The single core topic should be determined together with the patient and should not need to be newly agreed upon for each session but rather be clearly embedded in the overall treatment plan.

Topic list for the current session

It appears useful to have the patient *summarize the results of each therapy session* briefly in writing with the support of the therapist. These summaries should include the following aspects: What did the patient take from the session, and what was helpful? What remains unresolved, and what should be addressed in the next session? Which homework tasks were agreed upon until the next session? It is essential to repeatedly go over these important components and to collaboratively process the connection to the overall treatment plan.

Summarize the results of each therapy session

> **Assure the Following for All Homework Assignments Between Sessions**
>
> - Did the patient understand the approach?
> - Do they know, in concrete terms, what they are supposed to do?
> - Do they know why they are supposed to do that? Do they recognize the individual advantages, and understand the exercise to be an important interim step to achieving subjectively meaningful goals?

The tempo of the session may be decreased due to patients suffering from significant medication adverse effects, such as sedation or cognitive slowing.

4.3   How to Get Patients Into Treatment: The Engagement Phase

Engagement phase

Learned resistance

The engagement phase is described as the first part of treatment with the objective to initially get the patient into treatment. Particularly patients with chronic positive symptoms often show a full range of *learned resistance* to becoming involved in a therapeutic process. This does not refer to a pronounced mistrust due to current acute paranoid symptoms. Unfavorably learned relationship patterns to the family of origin or other important social contacts may hinder the development of a stable therapist–patient connection. The same is also true for previous negative illness-related treatment experiences. For example, patients frequently have had the experience that physicians are solely concerned with whether or not voices are heard, but are not interested in the content of the voices or the possible connection of this content to important personal experiences. Or patients may have learned that admitting to still hearing voices will result in an increase in medication with potentially greater side effects. In other words, patients may have learned that becoming involved in treatment is not only not rewarded but has rather adverse consequences.

Addressing ongoing paranoid symptoms

Addressing ongoing paranoid symptoms requires a specific focus on the insecurity of the patient, i.e., the therapeutic contact must be binding and regular. This includes timely availability of the therapist, clarity about the how and when of crisis contacts in case the patient is in acute distress, which other clinicians may act as back-up for the therapist, etc. In addition, the therapist's approach must be very transparent to the patient, i.e., the patient should be aware of the how and why of the collaborative approach. The patient's burdensome emotions of feeling badgered, agitated, and persecuted, as well as possible anger, despondency, or hopelessness regarding past experience, must be respectfully and appropriately addressed by means of supporting adequate coping attempts. Especially emotions subsequent to delusional misinterpretations must be the empathetic focus during this important phase of therapy in order to develop a working alliance with the patient.

Patients who hear voices

However, *patients who hear voices* may also present with substantial *resistance*. For many patients, discussing voices is associated with fears that the voices could become as aggressive, destructive, and invasive as during more acute phases of illness when the patient may have felt helpless and threatened, when the patient may have experienced traumatizing suicidality or forced hospitalizations or treatment. The patient's characteristic as "emotion avoider" may present here. Emotions very often influence preexisting cognitive disturbances, cause additional confusion and uncertainty, or become associated with the fear of a renewed massive exacerbation of the illness. An additional obstacle may be the previous patient experience of their doctors' failing to engage when patients began talking about delusional symptoms or hallucinations, but rather, simply and in a reflexive manner, increased neuroleptic medications with the risk of increased side effects.

Getting patients involved in cognitive behavioral treatment should, in general, be easier in *multiprofessional outpatient settings*, since the primary therapist – regardless of professional background – has often already been experienced as helpful for various reasons, e.g., help with financial difficulties, improvement of living situation, or reduction of medication side effects. Sometimes, however, it can be a disadvantage when the cognitive behavioral therapist is also responsible for forced therapeutic actions in the context of self-danger or danger to others, and for involuntary hospitalizations. In order not to damage the therapeutic relationship over the long term, primary therapists may decide to implement a *"good cop / bad cop" division of responsibilities* in which another team member initiates any necessary involuntary measures. However, it is by no means inevitable that the therapeutic relationship will suffer from such safety-related and required measures (Kingdon, 1998).

Many patients who have had unfavorable previous experiences with treatment must first become familiar with the different approach of CBT. In the cognitive therapy of positive symptomatology, the psychiatrist or psychotherapist must address the content of the psychotic symptoms, e.g., by asking, "What are the voices saying?" "How do you get the idea that…?" etc. Symptoms and associations based on learned experiences are not simply formally assessed, i.e., whether or not delusions or hallucinations are present (which is more than sufficient for a strict diagnostic classification and risk assessment).

In addition, fears of stigmatization can hinder the opening up of the patient: He or she may have experienced in their social environment but also with professional clinical contacts that, due to their acknowledgment of still existing or newly emerged psychotic symptoms, their self-image and self-esteem will come "under pressure." The patient may feel once again "mentally ill" and labeled as someone who is trusted less by the public due to stereotypes and stigma. For this reason, a longer initial treatment phase is frequently required before the patient will start to open up.

Naturally, an *unrealistically high expectation* of the patient and the *lack of immediate improvement on the symptom level* can make the start of treatment more difficult. Additionally, positive functions of persistent symptoms can prevent the patient from seeking treatment. Examples of this include cases in which voices served as a substitute for social contacts in the past, or delusional "explanations" served to justify past personal failure.

The building of *trust and security* is at the forefront of the initial therapeutic work. Not only are the bond and clarity of the therapeutic contact and the transparency of the approach of importance, but also conversational psychotherapeutic techniques such as empathy, verbalization of the content of emotional experience, as well as congruence.

Initial engagement may be more difficult for patients who are essentially socially withdrawn and live in isolation. At least initially, it is often necessary in such cases to reduce the length of sessions to 20–30 minutes in order not to overburden the patient (Kingdon, 1998). Furthermore, it is important for the development of the working alliance with the patient to engage in therapeutic conduct referred to as "befriending" which, for example, may include discussing hobbies or areas of interest with the patient, taking relaxed walks together, or offering a soda or coffee, and which generally aims to create a warm-hearted and relaxed environment. At the same time, nonverbal signals which may indicate mistrust or apprehension on the part of the patient must be acknowledged. The therapist should make these signals explicit, e.g., by asking questions such as "Have I done something that has displeased you?" etc. Again, normalizing can serve to stabilize the patient–clinician relationship and to guard against the fear of self-stigmatization (see also Section 4.4).

The term illness insight can lead to confusion

Sometimes the term *illness insight* can lead to confusion. It is important to emphasize that the CBT approach does not require insight. The patient does not have to have full illness insight and thus attribute his or her fears to delusional misperceptions or recognize delusions as delusions or the hearing of voices as auditory hallucinations, and both as the expressions of a psychotic illness. CBT does not require the patient to interpret delusional fears or voice hearing as "internally generated" disturbances of perception. This falls in line with the notion that illness insight is neither a necessary nor a sufficient requirement for patients taking medications (David, 1990). In other words, the simple willingness of patients to agree to regularly take neuroleptic medications is in no way based on the patient attributing all of his or her psychotic experiences to a mental illness. It would be more precise to think of the patient's *subjective illness and treatment theory*. It is important, however, that during the initial treatment phase, patients are led to a type of *view* that will motivate them to cooperate. Three case examples may illustrate this.

Patient's subjective illness and treatment theory

Illness Insight Is Not a Prerequisite for Cooperation

- A patient believes that evil forces are changing his or her thinking and that his or her brain is particularly susceptible to these influences during phases of insomnia. Here it would be sufficient if the patient were ready to try whether or not a sedating antipsychotic medication might help him reduce the subjective vulnerability felt during the night.

- When a patient assumes that voices are the expression of a mental illness and metabolic disturbances in the brain, but that this brain disease has been caused by aliens, the patient, strictly speaking does not have insight into the illness. Nevertheless, the therapist may be able to convince the patient that the initial goal is to weaken the destructive influence of the mental illness on the patient's life and to make himself "untouchable" using methods of modern medicine such as antipsychotic medication.

- Although a patient may no longer consider the occurrence of voices as the expressions of truly existing speech by invisible external persons, e.g., through walls or from the other side of the door, he or she may not necessarily have insight into the existence of a psychiatric illness. The patient may explain the occurrence of voices by postulating an external electrical energy which creates these pathologic phenomena. Nevertheless, insight into the deceptive character of the voices can facilitate engagement into therapy. The patient can more easily be moved into the important "observer role" from which he or she can view and explain favorable and unfavorable influences on his or her experience, as well as examine and test explanatory models in the therapy process using alternative explanations for symptoms.

When speaking of illness insight and its promotion, interventions should always target those changes in patients' subjective explanations for psychotic experiences that foster any minimal willingness to cooperate with the therapist. Insight-promoting strategies may be classified into three different groups (Nelson, 1997):

Strategies to Aid Insight

- Destigmatizing and normalizing
- Differentiating between experiences and facts using the cognitive model
- Making connections between the content of delusions and voices and the patient's biography and specific learning experiences

(Details regarding these individual interventions may be found in Section 4.4.)

The therapist should *not* try to replace a patient's inadequate subjective explanatory model regarding causes and change possibilities of the psychotic experience with the concept "This is my illness." Many patients reject this explanatory model due to feeling stigmatized by being labeled as having a mental illness and feeling worried that they will no longer be taken seriously by their therapists. One can possibly reach the patient with the explanation that others out of concern for him or her are conceptualizing his or her behavior as a possible expression of an illness.

4.4 Building a Stable Therapeutic Alliance

Some patients find that the *emotional risk of psychotherapy* is too high. They are afraid that they will become destabilized if they address negative feelings or disturbing residual symptoms. At the start of treatment, it is absolutely necessary to address the patient's fear of destabilization and related increases in symptoms and relapse risk. Additional obstacles to developing a successful alliance with a patient are summarized in Table 6.

Emotional risk of psychotherapy

Table 6. Common difficulties or obstacles in developing a collaborative working relationship

- The individual's feelings of hopelessness, despondency, and despair about recovery and treatment
- The nature of the psychotic phenomena, which may limit the development of trust
- The patient's caution or fear about discussing personal matters
- Stigma issues, such as fear of appearing "mad" or "dumb"
- Discomfort and unfamiliarity with therapy
- Therapy confirming a sense that recovery is not progressing as well as hoped
- Previous experiences of pain associated with trusting others
- Unpleasant or unhelpful therapeutic contacts in the past

Adapted from Herrmann-Doig, Maude, & Edwards (2003).

The development of a collaborative working relationship contains multiple goals (adapted from Herrmann-Doig et al., 2003):

- Establishing therapy as a clear and safe space
- Conducting the necessary diagnostic assessments
- Developing a case formulation based on the patient's presenting concerns
- Developing a collaborative working model with the patient that will serve as the foundation for the problem list and the treatment plan
- Facilitating the progress of therapy to each applicable next stage

A range of strategies exist that can help deepen or solidify the therapeutic relationship (see Table 7 for an overview). Patients must gain a concrete *perception of the working method* in therapy, what is expected of them, but also what they can expect from their therapist. The *frequency of sessions* should also be adapted to this goal, and, specifically in the initial phase of treatment, if possible, one to two sessions per week may be offered. In case of multiple symptoms or cognitive functional disturbances, three sessions with abbreviated session duration, e.g., 20 to 30 minutes per week, may be appropriate. The session frequency may have to be negotiated with patients who have led very secluded lives before beginning therapy. The habitual social withdrawal and passivity through loss of stimulation – e.g., loss of job and social relationships – is often further maintained due to the avoidance of symptom-provoking triggers in social situations.

For hard-to-engage patients, it may be of great advantage at first to only offer *practical support*, e.g., help with residential or financial issues. If the patient initially experiences the therapist as helpful in such practical areas, he or she is often more willing to engage in therapy based on the newly established trust. Once the patient is engaged, it is important to continuously root the patient in the therapeutic process throughout the course of treatment. This can be encouraged by having *interim treatment evaluations* to discuss with the patient what he or she has achieved to date and what the next required steps are to achieve personally meaningful goals. The potentially increasing awareness of the patient's own social decline and loss of important, familiar social relationships

Patients must gain a concrete perception of the working method

Frequency of sessions

Practical support

Interim treatment evaluations

Table 7. Strategies to solidify a therapeutic relationship

- Make the structure of treatment transparent, and clarify patient and therapist roles
- Explore and understand the patient's subjective working model of his or her difficulties and incorporate it respectfully
- Be an active listener; offer clarifications; when doing so, very carefully and sensitively address the patient's anxieties or persistent psychopathologic symptoms
- Every session should have concrete positive results for the patient and thus have him or her experience the philosophy of progress in small steps with subsequent encouragement
- Increase trust by offering interest in the patient himself, e.g., discuss the patient's hobbies and potentially plan joint activities at first until a relationship develops
- Continuously negotiate the length and frequency as well as the location of individual therapy sessions

such as family and friends, can complicate the course of therapy. This loss, in addition to the patient's *change of roles,* must also be properly *"mourned."*

The *working model* of patient and therapist develops in an interactive manner and requires the negotiation of professional and patient perspectives. In concrete terms, it is important to know the patient's *"subjective illness model"* and to develop an understanding of what the patient, and also the therapist, believes may have contributed to the initial development of the psychotic disturbance or to the relapse. Furthermore, the patient's ideas about factors maintaining psychotic symptoms must be processed. In this context, the significance of different forms of pharmacotherapy and CBT to the patient should be discussed. Finally, the roles of the patient and the therapist in the treatment process must be negotiated and clarified. The objective is for patients to develop an understanding of their current situation and at the same time to create the foundation for meaningful therapeutic target items and treatment modalities. It has been shown to be useful to capture the working model in written format for later reference. See example below (Herrmann-Doig, 2003):

> **Example of a Brief Patient Working Model**
>
> I have had many stressors in my life, and I have found it hard to cope with them. When I get very stressed these days, I hear voices. I have difficulty knowing how to respond to them, and it may be helpful for me to learn more effective ways to cope.

The so-called *normalizing approach* can be very helpful when developing the working model (Kingdon & Turkington, 2005). Here, analogies from daily experience are repeatedly used to explain psychotic experiences. For example, most patients are surprised and, at the same time, feel a sense of relief from shame and stigmatization fears, when they hear that every person can have psychotic experiences, such as hearing voices, after 2 to 3 days of sleep deprivation or after amphetamine injections. With such background knowledge, the patient may for the first time understand certain therapy strategies, such as the use of neuroleptic medications for the normalization of sleep patterns. An additional typical example is the use of the vulnerability–stress model to classify predispositions, triggers, and also perpetuating factors of the patient's illness. It can be very helpful here to use the example of a chronic medical illness as an analogy. Diabetes, for instance, presents with certain vulnerability factors such as a genetic predisposition, but also triggers such as pancreatitis or a viral infection, which can precede symptom exacerbation. At the same time, this is also an illness that requires both pharmacologic interventions, i.e., oral antidiabetics or insulin, as well as a change in lifestyle, e.g., healthy diet and exercise. It is also important to include the relevance of significant life events and life tasks as triggers, such as moving to a new home, starting or finishing school, or leaving the parental home.

At the end of this therapy phase, the goal should be the development of a *treatment plan,* including the precise listing of goals and partial goals, as well as the steps to achieve them. It is imperative to involve the suggestions and wishes of the patient. It can be difficult with some patients to build up sufficient problem insight, because of impairment by negative symptoms such as passivity, or due to their denial of the existence of any problems.

If the therapist perceives resistance to therapy in general or with regard to a specific goal, this resistance should be addressed directly and clarified (see example below) (Safran & Muran, 2000). That should be done in question format as if testing a work hypothesis: "Could it be that it is difficult for you…. and consequently you always … when …?" Consequently, the patient feels better understood, and thus this type of approach will help stabilize the therapeutic relationship.

It may be possible that, due to cognitive impairment, the patient is not clear about the motivating reasons for his or her resistance to treatment or to specific therapy aspects. Attentional impairment ("What is most important?") and memory problems ("What was my previous situation like, and how will my future situation be?") often prevent the patient from recognizing the need and opportunity for a therapeutic intervention. Also, deficits in working memory may hinder the ability for self-observation and consequently the recognition of problems and impairments. Disability or psychotic relapses and crises due to career failure and failure in social relationships frequently threaten the identity of the adult patient. Therefore, patients can experience the "obligation" to therapy as an additional threat to their autonomy. An example of how to respond as a therapist is described below.

Therapist: You always seem a bit as though I must convince you to really come to treatment following your release from inpatient care. Is that correct?

Patient: Yes, my physician in the hospital said I should stop by your place.

Therapist: I assume that you have reasons for why you are so reluctant and doubt that this is the right thing for you. Perhaps it would be helpful for me to get to know these feelings so that I can better understand your reluctance?

Other examples of how a therapist could react, include:

- "I do not know exactly what is troubling you, but for many people in your situation it is not easy to commit to follow-up treatment because they often think that a guard has been assigned to them because others don't trust that they can go on with their own lives. Is this perhaps a reason that applies to you?"

- "I have the impression that you are trying very hard to be a normal young man and not to differentiate yourself from other students your age. You would like to forget the illness, the burdensome symptoms, to have as little to do with them as possible, so that you can feel like your friends as quickly as possible. Is that correct?"

- "Sometimes people who have lived through psychotic experiences during a crisis have the strong desire to simply forget the illness and to give it as little space in their own lives as possible. For some it can then be scary to confront in psychotherapy past psychotic experiences which were very stressful."

- "Oftentimes the fear or concern plays a role that these symptoms may increase or reappear, if one discusses them in therapy. Is this the case for you?"

Follow up with:

- "Would it then be possible to try … ?" [offer alternatives which protect the wish/need of the patient]
- "Is it always the case that if …, then …?"

Frequently the assignment of patients to CBT in outpatient clinics is organized by inpatient staff arranging follow-up care after a hospitalization due to a recent acute exacerbation of symptoms. Alternatively, relatives, who often bear a substantial psychological strain themselves, initiate treatment for their affected family member. In these cases, it is very important to clarify the motivation for treatment with the patient at the outset of the therapeutic process.

Typical *Initial Questions* to Clarify Personal Versus External Motivation for Treatment

"You are coming to our treatment center. What does your physician/relative say is the problem? ... Do you agree? ... What do you yourself think is the trouble? ... Is there also something that you wish to achieve for yourself?"

Initial Questions

If a patient has been treated *nonspecifically over a very long time* in general outpatient services, and a treatment course of illness- and problem-specific CBT is initiated as a possible chance for symptom improvement, the therapist may frequently struggle with a full range of difficulties which are summarized in Table 8.

The successful engagement of the patient in therapy is often hindered in several ways. Patients often fear – e.g., when talking about voices – that those then become more intense, more aggressive, or louder so that another inpatient admission is unavoidable (catastrophic thinking). By repeated attempts to avoid psychotic experiences, the patient may be able to achieve a short-term reduction in fear, but an increased occurrence of voice hearing and also delusional fears may follow. These intrusion-like experiences, as well as actual acute symptom exacerbation, increase the feeling of loss of control. Patients may conclude that they are helpless when facing psychotic experiences, e.g., that the voices are omnipotent. This pattern of confrontation avoidance and failure-oriented thinking at the start of treatment is therefore a very important obstacle for engagement into the treatment process.

Table 8. Obstacles to treatment motivation prior to initiation of cognitive behavioral therapy for voice hearing and delusions

- Fear to begin focusing on psychotic symptoms, out of concern that these may then become stronger, less controllable, etc.
- Impairments in concentration or other cognitive functions which make participation in therapy difficult
- Reluctance to be seen as ill
- Psychotic symptoms as justification for life choices (If the voices/pursuer did not exist, then ...); mistrust toward the anticipated medical model (stereotyped thinking, stigmatization fears, experiences of involuntary hospitalization, or increase in side effects with higher dose of medications)
- Mistrust/hostile interpersonal style (previous learning experience, early bonding, paranoid symptoms themselves)
- Comorbidity (in particular addiction)
- Experience that personal life events, previous learning experiences, and individual characteristics are not taken seriously enough in therapy
- Hasty, confrontational approach of the therapist

Many patients have had unfavorable treatment experiences

In addition to these symptom-specific expectational fears and a generalized tendency to avoid being overburdened, many patients have had *unfavorable treatment experiences,* including involuntary hospitalizations and medication increases, as outlined above. While such treatment measures may very well have been indicated to guarantee the safety of the patient and others, they may lead to resistance to treatment, to an increase in internally generated stigma, and to related concerns that one is considered once again as ill and incapable of living. This self-stigmatization is frequently reinforced by the environment, creating a vicious circle: Because the patient does not seek treatment, often very critical situations arise in which relatives and/or caretakers must then react very quickly for the significantly impaired patient, which confirms the feeling of inability to live independently and consequently reproduces the social reality of stigma and high levels of expressed emotion in the overburdened social surrounding.

Again, the *normalizing* approach (Kingdon & Turkington, 2005) can be very helpful for correcting the catastrophic thinking of the patient ("I am an incurable sick person"). *Normalizing* does not, however, mean "minimizing." By normalizing symptoms, patients may also learn the significance of proper coping techniques for these challenges. For instance, they may learn that social withdrawal can intensify psychotic symptoms such as voices and brooding about delusional insecurities. By learning to connect voices and delusions with important previous life events, their experiences can become more understandable and less anxiety producing so that misattribution and self-stigmatization are decreased.

Therapy always and continuously means taking an emotional risk

Patient must feel safe in the therapeutic working relationship

In response to "hesitation" to engage, the patient must at first perceive acceptance and a pressure-free attitude. The therapist has to acknowledge that therapy always and continuously means *taking an emotional risk* for the patient. Similar to other exposure and response prevention approaches, patients must have control over when to bring up psychotic experiences in therapy. Again and again it is emphasized that opening up is voluntary and that the patient should maintain control of this decision. Another essential prerequisite is that the patient must *feel safe in the therapeutic working relationship and trust the therapist.*

Partnership-based guidance of the patient

Partnership-based guidance of the patient instead of a paternalistic approach encourages the development of a more efficient therapeutic alliance. The therapist must be aware that the acute phase, which often requires substantial disregard of patient wishes to assure patient safety, can never serve as a model for treatment in the maintenance phase. It is necessary to continuously encourage the patient's motivation for equal contributions and thus foster the sharing of responsibilities in the therapy process. This may mean accepting differential perspectives regarding goals and approaches to the treatment process. To achieve this, it is necessary to thoroughly process the *individual advantages and disadvantages* of specific treatment options with the patient and thereby emphasize his or her own individual responsibility.

Principle of collaborative empiricism

The formation of a therapeutic relationship based on the principle of *collaborative empiricism* also involves partnership-based patient guidance. The patient's experiences are examined collaboratively to check whether they justify the patient's assessments and should confirm his or her fears. The therapist repeatedly stresses that it can be helpful to closely examine personal experiences and related life events and learning experiences. Gaining an understanding of such connections can provide clarity and reduce stress for the patient, as illustrated in the following example: A patient associates the neighbor's voice asking him to move, with the experience of an involuntary admission to a hospital. Through work in session, the patient then understands that a neighbor contacted the police only because of the patient's ongoing loud music, which was the patient's reaction to his or her own florid psychotic symptoms.

The patient's illness-related knowledge, i.e., subjective illness theory and treatment expectations, should also be processed using this principle of collaborative empiricism. The patient's theory and expectations should be the basis for each psychoeducation exercise, and only later should other materials be used in a targeted manner.

4.5 Special Aspects of Patient Treatment for Chronic Positive Symptoms

Depending on how severely a patient's *cognitive impairment or psychotic symptoms* interfere with therapy, it can make the most sense to see the patient more frequently for briefer sessions (e.g., 30 min twice a week instead of once for 50 min) (Haddock & Tarrier, 1998). For the same reason, communication should be kept very clear, and the processing of excessively complex or ambiguous issues should be delayed.

Cognitive impairment or psychotic symptoms interfere

In general, individual therapy should be supplemented with *family therapy interventions*, i.e., family psychoeducation and support for problem-solving in the family, if the patient has regular contact with his or her relatives. The goal is to reduce high levels of expressed emotion communication patterns, which

Family therapy interventions

Table 9. Risk factors for suicide in psychotic patients
• Young and male
• Unmarried
• Unemployed
• Past history of suicide attempts
• Family history of suicide
• Family stress or instability
• Recent loss or rejection
• Limited external support
• Depression, depressed mood, or sense of hopelessness
• Good premorbid functioning prior to a chronic illness with numerous exacerbations, and high levels of psychopathology and functional impairment
• Realistic awareness of deteriorative effects of illness and fear of further mental deterioration
• Excessive treatment dependence or loss of faith in treatment
Adapted from Haddock & Tarrier (1998)

often result from the overburden of the relatives, but can double the chances of relapse (Hahlweg, 2006), see also Chapter 1.2.

Finally, it should be noted that life events frequently represent triggers for relapse and the worsening of symptoms for people with psychotic disorders. Consequently, foreseeable significant life changes, such as moving, beginning or ending of school or employment, etc., should be planned well in advance, if possible. Controllable life events should therefore be free of time pressure and planned systematically together with the patient. Increased therapeutic support during such times should also be offered, i.e., an increase in session frequency.

Suicidal risk assessments

Suicidal risk assessments in cases of chronic positive symptoms should be completed regularly since the lifetime risk for completed suicides is approximately 10% to 12%. Frequent risk factors are listed in Table 9.

A particular difficulty in the treatment of delusional patients is that often very early on they pressure the therapist to agree with them with regard to their assumed delusional contents, e.g., feelings of being followed. Here the use of nondirective conversational strategies and statements such as "I must learn more before I can agree with you," "I see that you are very sure about this," or "At present I am not sure; however, I like listening to you" have been proven to be helpful (Kingdon, 1998).

5 Cognitive Behavioral Therapy Strategies for Chronic Voice Hearing

5.1 Reduction of Fear and Increase of Control: Focusing Techniques

Focusing techniques include a variety of different interventions that guide the patient in the self-confrontation with voice hearing. Generally, this refers to patients learning to gradually turn their attention toward the internal experiences of hearing voices (Haddock, Slade, Bentall, Reid, & Faragher, 1998). The goal is for patients to adopt the role of an observer and consequently identify increasingly more details about the voices and to learn to better distance themselves emotionally from the voices. Through decreased avoidance of confrontations with the voices, patients will experience fewer feelings of *loss of control (expectancy anxiety)* and uncontrolled breakthrough psychotic experiences (*intrusions*).

Focusing techniques

Fewer feelings of loss of control

Table 10. Example of initiating questions for work on symptom and coping diaries

Triggers	Behavior	Consequences
• What thoughts/images went through your mind?	• *Characteristics* of the voice: How loud is it? Does it have an accent? Is it male or female? Where does it come from?	• *Behavior:* interference (What do you no longer do because of the voices?); coping (What do you do instead?)
• What *feelings* did you experience, e.g., mistrust, loss of control?	• *Content:* What exactly did the voice say?	• *Cognition:* possible delusional explanations and patient's evidence (How do you explain what the voices are saying?)
• What *were* you *doing* before the voices appeared?	• *Evaluation:* Do you feel in control of the voices or at their mercy? Do you experience the voice as friendly or hostile?	• *Effects on self image:* self-worth, expectations for controlling the voices
• *What were other people doing?*	• If applicable, explore any connection with *life experiences:* Do you recognize the voices from somewhere? The theme of what the voices are saying appears to be ... – do you know that from any area in your life?	• *Emotions*
• Are there internal or external *situations in which the voices are less stressful?*		

Gathering of information relevant for treatment planning

Generally speaking, the *gathering of information relevant for treatment planning* is already considered a type of focusing technique. Usually such information is gathered using three strategies:

(1) *voice hearing interviews*, see Appendices 1–3
(2) clinical exploration by means of a *symptom diary* or
(3) *during therapist-guided in sensu or in vivo symptom clarifications.*

Behavior- and environment-specific information

The last includes imagery exercises and the joint experiencing of voice-provoking situations with the goal of gathering *behavior- and environment-specific information* related to voice hearing. During an imagery exercise, the therapist may, for instance ask: "Please imagine the last situation in which you heard particularly intense stressful voices. Could we slowly examine them together?" Table 10 introduces a protocol for initiating questions when working on symptom and coping diaries.

What follows is an example dialogue based on Romme and Escher (2000), which also addresses the connection between voice content and core therapy themes relative to previous life experiences and past learning behavior.

Therapist: Did I understand that correctly that you are reluctant to discuss the voices because you are afraid they could become more aggressive?

Patient: Yes.

Therapist: Are you willing to take this risk here in session where you feel very safe?

Patient: What would you want to know?

Therapist: How loud is the voice? Is it precisely as loud as my voice or softer or louder? ... Does it come from outside your head, or does it rather come from inside? ... Is it male or female? ... You don't know exactly, so should we take a look at your voice diary together? ... I don't think it is actually that easy to remember correctly.... Do you still recall any particular situation during the past week in which you felt especially stressed by hearing the voice?

Patient: Yes, it happened when I woke up in the middle of the night, and the voices told me that my husband was possessed by the devil and would harm my 4-year-old son.

Therapist: Are you able to tell me *exactly* what the voices said? ... How did you feel at that time?

Patient: I was very afraid for my son.

Therapist: Were you afraid that your husband could physically injure your son?

Patient: Yes.

Therapist: Has your husband ever hit your son?

Patient: No, but he yells at him from time to time when he is impatient.

Therapist: And what do you think when your husband acts this way around you?

Patient: It aggravates me; I somehow find myself between the two of them.

Therapist: That is to say that it makes you nervous when your husband acts so impatiently with your son. Is that right?

Patient: Yes.

Therapist: Okay, that means that the voices express in a very extreme fashion a fear that you also have in everyday life. Is that correct? ... Do you know this also from other examples that the voices drastically express your fears, currently or in the past? ...

Other possibilities of focusing strategies include patients recording the content of the voices using a tape recorder. Should the voice content be very fear-inducing, then this can be done in the presence of the therapist. Also, patients can share the content of the voices with the therapist in session as they are experienced. The therapist can teach the patient to concentrate on the voices and to perhaps allow them to become louder (*focusing*) and then to concentrate again on a relaxing, safer situation (imagery). This type of *distancing* corresponds to the well-known *change of focus to an "internal safe place"* used in the self-confrontation therapy of posttraumatic stress disorder. Another option for distancing is the use of *mindfulness exercises* from dialectic-behavioral therapy of borderline personality disorder. Here, the patient learns to concentrate on an action (e.g., rinse cycle when doing dishes) or an object (e.g., a cup of hot coffee) using all senses and initially to verbally describe the experience to the therapist: "I feel the pleasant warmth of the full cup of coffee in my hand, smell the aroma of coffee and taste the slightly bitter coffee when drinking it," etc. (for details, see Eickhoff, Vauth, & Olbrich, 1997; Linehan, 1993). It is important for all of these exercises that the confrontation of the voices happens in a phased manner depending on the extent to which negative feelings are induced by the process, e.g., fear. The focusing exercise should be interrupted before the fear becomes unbearable for the patient, so that the patient strengthens his or her feeling of control and does not experience defeat. The study by Haddock et al. (1998) showed that a therapy approach including self-confrontation strategies such as focusing exercises can increase self-esteem to a greater extent than learning pure distraction strategies.

Change of focus to an "internal safe place"

Mindfulness exercises

5.2 Change of Evaluative Processes for Voice Hearing

The patient's reaction to voice hearing sometimes already allows speculations regarding possible *evaluative processes*. If the patient, for instance, actively listens to the voices, is willing to follow their suggestions (compliance with the voices), and also does things to make the voices occur more often – e.g., creates situations in which the voices appear more frequently, such as turning on the television – one can assume that the voices are most likely considered *benevolent* or *helpful*. If the patient, however, shows open or concealed resistance to the voices, e.g., he argues with them or even yells in order to drown them out, then the voices are often considered *malevolent*. In these cases, treatment compliance may only happen under extreme pressure, and trigger situations are generally avoided. If no clear relationship pattern with the voice exists, indifferent behavior is most likely.

Evaluative processes

The *clarification of the patient's "relationship" to the voices* is a very important process. The therapist coaches the patient to enter into an open dialogue with the voices, e.g., by recording the voices, as discussed above. This allows the *joint listening to the "voice protocol"* and immediate cognitive work with the content. When discussing the voices' content, therapists frequently introduce two analogies:

Clarification of the patient's "relationship" to the voices

(1) The All-Knowing Expert
   The voices take it upon themselves to always know what is best and right for the life of the patient and to apparently be able to objectively

assess the patient. Similar to experts, they do not clarify the background of their evaluations and consequently gain an omnipotent role for the patient.

(2) The Evil Neighbor

The voices act just like a bad neighbor who makes rude comments across the fence.

By means of these didactic analogies, the therapist tries to awaken a willingness in the patient to take a critical look at the content of the voices. The following text box gives an example of the types of questions used in this coaching process.

Example of Socratic Questioning for Patient Training on Questioning Negative Voice Content

- Is it actually true that you, like the voice is accusing you, always/never do … ?
- Is it actually true that you, like the voice is accusing you, always/never are … ?
- Does this correspond with your personal experiences?
- Or are there also counterexamples?
- Can you explain this to me in more detail?
- In your opinion, is there evidence for …, that is so plausible that it would hold up in court because it is objectively verifiable and reasonable?

The questioning of voice contents by means of Socratic questioning or the gathering of evidence to support or contradict voice content represents important strategies to triumph over the feeling of helplessness caused by voice hearing.

The patient learns to critically question the "arrogant expert" or "evil neighbor" – e.g., "What exactly does this actually mean what you are telling me again? What exactly do you mean by this?" Throughout this process, the therapist will repeatedly use psychoeducational elements, e.g., developing a *vicious cycle model* together with the patient. Within the context of the model and based on patients' own words and experiences, patients should realize the following: By distracting themselves from hearing the voices, by avoiding them or by being subservient to them, they repeatedly experience a lack of control. Consequently, the trust and confidence in their ability to handle the voices successfully is continuously weakened. In the frequent scenario of patients expe-

Developing a vicious cycle model together with the patient

Coleman, a voice hearer himself, provides an example of the importance of cognitive restructuring (Coleman & Smith, 2003, p. 26):

"I would, for example, ask a voice hearer who receives the order from his voices to kill himself, to question his voices as to why they are requesting this, and to encourage him to demand an answer. One cannot let the voices get away with replies such as 'You deserve it' or 'You are evil.' You need a real explanation. Don't forget: You have the right to say no! … If your convictions are founded on telepathy then you are also saying that you have a special gift. If this is the case, you most likely have other talents as well … and [can] build a wall in your mind that does not allow the negative thoughts to pass through. You will probably need some endurance to achieve this; however, it is worthwhile to learn it."

riencing concentration difficulties and working memory impairments, it may be helpful to briefly record the counterarguments with the help of the therapist, e.g., against specific accusations by the voices. In doing so, helpful evaluations / alternative explanations will be available to the patient also outside the therapy session.

5.3 Improving Coping Strategies

Tarrier's coping strategy enhancement (CSE) approach (Tarrier et al., 1993) assumes that the patient's avoidance behavior maintains the fear of the voices and the feeling of inferiority to the voices by weakening the trust in individual coping abilities. In his approach, Tarrier therefore differentiates between a diagnostic, a motivational, and an intervention phase. The purpose of the diagnostic phase is to complete a problem analysis based on behavioral therapy principles. In addition to trigger and behavior analyses, this also includes the evaluations of the voices and associated possible consequences (see Table 10). In the analysis of *spontaneous coping strategies,* physical, cognitive, and behavior-based techniques are differentiated, and their short- and long-term consequences as well as their effectiveness are recorded. An example of a possible self-observation protocol can be found in Table 11.

Tarrier emphasizes the need to not solely rely on verbal statements made by the patient, but he stresses the importance of addressing emotionally charged evaluation processes (so-called "hot cognitions") rather than simply assessing the patient's rationalizing thoughts, i.e., what the patient believes and thinks about the voices. This can be achieved by either collaboratively working through a *voice-provoking trigger situation* or by means of *imagery exercises.* People with psychotic disorders are often very imprecise in their verbal self-statements because of their cognitive limitations. If the therapeutic process is based on such *inaccuracies* or *rationalizations,* then therapy can set completely incorrect focal points for treatment. Therefore, it is important to ask exactly what it is that makes the patient fearful or angry. As discussed in the previous

Table 11. Example of a self-observation protocol to improve spontaneous coping strategies

Weekday/ Time	Triggers: What did I do? What about others?	Content: What did the voices say?	Reaction: What did I do / attempt to do?	Ameliorating factors/ behaviors: What can make the voices less destructive/ burdensome?	Perpetuating factors/ behaviors: What can make the voices worse?
Tuesday, 11/15	Riding the bus.	Nothing will ever become of you!	Turned on portable disc player.	Instead of music, listen to a book on tape.	If my mood was already bad prior to the voices.

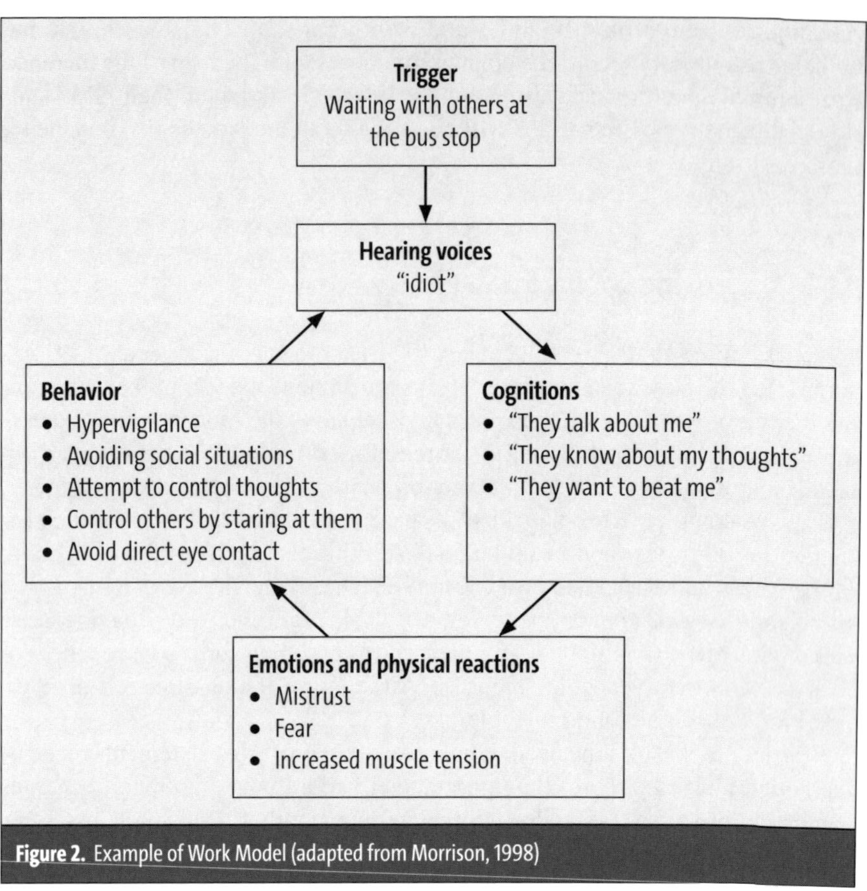

Figure 2. Example of Work Model (adapted from Morrison, 1998)

section, it is important also to investigate schemas relative to previous life experiences that may be a foundation for the content of the voices, as well as to identify relevant past learning behaviors that may be precursors to some of the voice content. The goal is to help the patient develop new evaluations of voice hearing which in turn will make the patient feel "liberated." As *a result of the diagnostic phase,* the patient and the therapist develop a joint work model that investigates which vicious circles maintain the emotional burden caused by hearing voices. Diagnostic elements and psychoeducation alternate during this phase. During this time, it is also important to explain the role of any avoidance behavior as a chronicity factor. An example for this type of work model is shown in Figure 2.

Result of the diagnostic phase

The *second phase, the motivational phase,* of CSE primarily focuses on a functional analysis of persistent psychotic behavior. The central question is, what advantages could the patient gain from better mastering the voices and from feeling less dominated by them? Could there also be disadvantages? It is important for the clinician to remember that seemingly positive changes in the evaluation process of voice hearing could also have disadvantages for self-evaluative processes – e.g., personal failure is attributed to voice hearing.

Motivational phase

In the *third phase*, the actual *intervention phase*, of CSE, patients practice the initial use or more effective use of existing effective and socially tolerable coping strategies based on the patient's preexisting self-help repertoire. This can occur based on spontaneous manifestations of voice hearing in the therapy

Intervention phase

session, based on audiotape protocols of voice content recorded by the patient, or based on role plays analogous to the two-chair technique from behavioral therapy where the concealed internal dialogue with the voice is changed to an external dialogue. It is important for the therapist to maintain a gradual change from less threatening to more threatening voice content and to continuously evaluate whether the patient subjectively experiences success – e.g., a decrease of the emotional impairment or the distraction caused by the voices. It can also be important to first practice the strategies, such as distraction or relaxation, outside the actual therapeutic target before implementing it for voice hearing.

For the therapeutic implementation of spontaneous coping behavior, it is very important to move patients to voluntarily relinquish cognitive or behavioral *avoidance behaviors*. This work is analogous to response prevention in the treatment of obsessive-compulsive disorder.

Avoidance behaviors

A large number of coping strategies are available to cope with voice hearing. They are presented in Table 12 (see also Appendix: Strategy Card – Voice Hearing).

Table 12. Overview of coping strategies for voice hearing

Reduction of tension
- Coping cue cards: "Stay calm," "Think this through," "Am I jumping to conclusions?"
- Relaxation: progressive muscle relaxation or similar strategies

Distraction methods
- Headphones for active listening to music
- Ear plugs (for voices)
- Reading aloud
- Humming or singing out loud or to self
- Exercise
- Concentrating on the radio or television
- Ignoring the voices
- Talking to others
- Sleeping
- Concentrating on naming and describing objects in the room – out loud or to self

Focusing methods
- Observing and describing the voices – tone, content, gender, etc. – and their meaning and relationship with thoughts and beliefs
- "Bringing on" the voices in sessions with the therapist and using strategies to minimize distress and symptoms
- Graded exposure to feared situations, preferably with the help of the therapist

Other methods
- Activity scheduling
- If I am not sure about what I am hearing and whether these are hallucinations or not, I can ask people in whom I have confidence whether they can hear what I am hearing

Adapted from Herrmann-Doig, Maude, & Edwards (2003)

Try different strategies over a long period

While working on improving a patient's coping repertoire, clinicians must remember that the patient may already have experienced a substantial amount of failure. Patients must be *prepared that they may have to try different strategies over a long period of time* and will notice improvement only gradually and only after a while. Consequently, Coleman includes the following important message in his workbook for patients (Coleman & Smith, 2003, p. 5):

> We cannot, and do not stress enough in this book that this work is ongoing and hard and at first you may not find the coping strategies immediately working.
>
> It's OK when things don't work!!!
>
> They will in the long run, if not directly, by giving you the energy to look at the way you see the voices and understand them. From this you can try new ways and think of your own by moving from the *victim to the victor*.

Distraction strategies

Distraction strategies are based on the knowledge that only a limited amount of information can be processed simultaneously. Thus, creating information competition with the voices by the patient is a very effective strategy to weaken the influence of the voices. The temporary wearing of one earplug leads to the open ear, the contralateral ear, having to "compensate" for the information meant to be processed by the closed ear. Consequently, attention is oriented more toward the outside, and by means of this strong "exterior orientation," attention to the inside and what the voices are saying is reduced. Usually, this technique can only be used if voices present temporary "peaks" in intensity. If earplugs are worn for a longer period of time (approx. 15–30 min), habituation occurs, and consequently, information competition with voice content becomes more limited. Another option is the use of headphones so the patient concentrates on music, or better to audio books (because of similarities to voices). This principle of information competition is used successfully as the "shadowing" technique in the treatment of tinnitus.

Case Example for Walkman/Discman and iPod Use

A patient who had been suffering from voice hearing for a very long time despite high-dosage clozapine treatment, was barely able to leave his apartment and use public transportation to attend a therapeutic workshop and his outpatient therapist. When rides on public transit lasted longer than 10 minutes and many other passengers were present, the voices became extremely aggressive and loud. This was so agonizing that the patient could only stand this state for a few minutes before having to put an end to the situation and having to leave, e.g., getting off at the next stop. A consequence of this was that he could not keep steady employment nor could he systematically and consistently engage in psychotherapy. At the same time, his self-esteem weakened and his feeling of powerlessness over the voices became stronger.

Now, the patient was very interested in soccer and listened to the soccer radio reports every Saturday afternoon. The therapist and patient agreed that the patient would regularly record these soccer reports on audio cassettes in order to play them on his Walkman while using public transportation. The result was that the patient concentrated in a targeted manner on information that was emotionally attractive to him (soccer reports), thereby substantially weakening the influence of the aggressive voices. This distraction method was effective, similar to tinnitus masking, primarily because listening to soccer reports was *an emotionally*

> *positive experience for the patient.* By using this self-help strategy, the patient was able to use public transportation for up to 2 hours, including during the heaviest commuting periods. This increased his feeling of control over the voices and generally the feeling of regaining control over his life (self-efficacy, empowerment). At the same time, this coping experience weakened the expectancy fears ("I will not make it again this time since the voices are too loud and I cannot stand it"), which generally occurred at the beginning of a trip using public transportation.

Humming and singing can also be a very effective masking strategy, due again in part to information competition. Studies have shown that the larynx muscle is innervated during the appearance of auditory hallucinations (Carter, Mackinnon, & Copolov, 1996). Neurobiological research has proven that humming or singing promotes the release of "endogenous morphine" (endorphin) (Kreutz, Bongard, Rohrmann, Hodapp, & Grebe, 2004), and consequently, mood ratings can improve during voice hearing. This appears to be a very effective strategy especially considering that depressed patients in schizodepressive episodes appear more at the mercy of voices than at times when moods are more balanced. Other distraction strategies, such as playing games, or getting in touch with social supporters (e.g., telephone calls) have been effective for some patients.

> **Humming and singing**

It has been shown for some patients that the appearance of voices is closely associated with states of high tension. These are often caused by stressful events such as family conflict or time pressure at work, by negative moods such as aggravation, fear, or anger, and also by strong physical stimulation such as shopping trips in congested areas with many pedestrians or in large department stores with additional sensory input like background music and significant visual stimulation. If a *clear connection exists between an increase in tension and an increase in voice hearing,* such as an increase in aggressive voice content, the practice of strategies to reduce tension can be very helpful. Specifically, progressive muscle relaxation (PMR) has been shown to be very effective. For chronic voice hearers, PMR has four goals:

> **Clear connection exists between an increase in tension and an increase in voice hearing**

(1)   Reduction of tension,
(2)   Improvement of self-perception,
(3)   Development of better symptom control, and consequently
(4)   Self-efficacy.

Besides reduction of tension, PMR is also helpful in the training of physical self-perception that is often limited in schizophrenia patients – i.e., the improved self-monitoring of physical signals of increased tension. The latter occurs precisely because PMR explicitly emphasizes and focuses on the differences between states of relaxation and states of tension. Thus, the patient learns self-instructions such as "I can really feel the tension in my muscles.... I can feel how all excessive tension is disappearing, and how I gain time to gather new energy...." Patients frequently suffer from feelings of loss of control and heteronomy due to voice hearing. The systematic induction of controlled muscular tension during PMR training can provide *feelings of being in control and safe,* which can be increased depending on the type of PMR script used and by employing the "safe place" technique, e.g., "I am sitting safely and firmly in my chair and feel how the back rest supports my back. My feet are planted

> **PMR training can provide feelings of being in control and safe**

firmly on the floor, etc." Since many avoidance behaviors are justified by the patient's desire for safety, the detailed imagery work on a "safe place" can be used as an alternative to avoidance, thereby undermining the vicious circle of illness chronicity. The following statements about voice hearing illustrate how important it is for patients to develop feelings of control (Splitter, 2003):

> The goal is to accept the voices as "internal companion" and to become the "master of his own home" again, and to become a "self-confident opponent" to the voices.

> Maybe it is the voices – they have made me into a powerful woman. Yes, at some point in time, I decided to stop being a victim. At some point, I had had enough. The all-powerful fear is gone. The voices can no longer cause me fear.

To warrant a successful transfer of skills to everyday situations, these strategies will have to be practiced in a targeted manner in possible real-life circumstances, preferably accompanied by the clinician. If a patient was able to be in a department store for 30 minutes before the voices became highly aversive, he or she will now learn to seek out a peaceful location in the vicinity of the shopping center after only 20 minutes, such as a quiet courtyard, a church, or the restroom of the shopping center. Once in this stimulus-controlled environment, patients then train themselves to close their eyes and possibly cover their ears and to imagine relaxing situations in which they feel safe and secure.

Practice of extended exhalation

A useful add-on technique is the practice of *extended exhalation*. An example script is: "You will exhale for twice as long as you will inhale. When you exhale, you will use the 'lip brake' in order to allow the air to escape very, very slowly." By means of extended exhalation, the parasympathetic nervous system becomes maximally stimulated, which works in opposition to the sympathetic nervous system, the mediator for stress reactions. Patients with difficulties in self-perception and correct execution of PMR techniques and extended exhalation can further benefit from individual biofeedback therapy, which uses measures such as heart rate and skin conductance to give patients real-life feedback for their physiological increase in tension and successful relaxation, via acoustic and visual feedback signals.

6 Cognitive Behavioral Therapy Strategies for Chronic Delusions

6.1 Creating the Right Conditions for Change: Normalizing and Using Analogies

Necessary prerequisites for successful cognitive work with delusional content include the normalizing of experiences, an explanation of the cognitive model, respectful dealings with the emotional consequences of delusional misinterpretations, and the practice of collaborative empiricism.

Clinicians can foster destigmatization by means of *normalizing* when explaining that delusional convictions do not differ qualitatively from normal psychological experiences, but merely quantitatively. In this context, psychoeducation works with two themes:

(a) the cognitive model, including the concept of typical cognitive distortions in everyday thinking and

(b) the two-pronged model of behavior control.

The hope in both approaches is that patients do not feel stigmatized and do not internalize negative stereotypes (self-stigmatization), therefore decreasing their self-esteem or potentially becoming reactionary, leading to disengagement from therapy due to feeling misunderstood. *Psychoeducation about typical cognitive distortions* in everyday thoughts should clarify that there are *no qualitative differences* between emotionally relevant belief systems with delusional content and those with nondelusional content, i.e., attitudes, evaluations, and conclusions.

In the case of delusional thought content, common psychological distortion tendencies simply occur in "accentuated" form. Examples include the tendency to process conforming schematic information faster and to favor this information during perception and memory processes (*conformation bias*), and the use of self-esteem benefiting statements for the interpretation of successes and failures (*self-serving bias*). Beck's *cognitive distortions* are viewed as valid in cases of delusional symptoms, such as all-or-nothing thinking, black-and-white thinking, or jumping to conclusions based on minimal initial information (Morrison, 1998). These are often combined with other types of cognitive distortions such as *over-generalizations of danger* (see Table 13) that are also typical for posttraumatic stress disorder (Ehlers, 1999; Eickhoff et al., 1997).

A second variation of the normalizing approach is the psychoeducational introduction of the so-called *two-pronged model of behavior control* (Nelson, 1997), explaining to the patient that on the one hand we have an automated, rather emotionally guided system of behavior regulation, and on the other hand,

Table 13. Typical errors in reasoning in the overgeneralization of danger	
Emotional reasoning	"I am so anxious; consequently there must be danger."
Seeing connections between independent events	"If everyone is staring at me at the bus stop and the bus driver also wants me to show my monthly pass, then this can only mean that everyone is out to give me a hard time."
Overgeneralization	"Danger lurks everywhere; I am too trusting."
Selective attention (hypervigilance)	"Someone is eavesdropping behind every tree."
Adapted from Ehlers (1999).	

we also have a rational system, which uses logical reasoning. Both the advantages and disadvantages of the two systems should be explained to the patient.

For example, clinicians might emphasize that evolutionarily speaking, the faster emotionally guided and automatic system created massive survival advantages during many acutely threatening situations. The advantage of the rational system based on logical reasoning consists in not needing to accept any initial behavioral and explanatory option, but rather to be able to test in a more targeted manner what is truly appropriate for the situation, the individual person, and one's own goals. The rational system is less prone to errors; however, it requires more time. The reason for introducing this analogy is to communicate to patients experiencing persistent delusions that their *conclusions are strongly guided by emotions*. This explanation is much more approachable for the patient than the more biological concept that the patient's fears are an expression of his or her illness which is, in turn, based on a metabolic disorder. It is frequently very difficult for patients to accept the presence of a mental illness, often based on the concerns that others will minimize or belittle their anxieties and fears, so they will end up stigmatized. Patients may be afraid that higher doses of antipsychotics used in an attempt to control the persistent delusions might bring on more severe side effects, and that patients might have to be hospitalized or otherwise treated against their will.

The starting point of cognitive restructuring is a *clear understanding of the cognitive model*. Patients must clearly understand that events (triggers = A) do not have immediate consequences (C). They must understand that it is the evaluation process (B) that causes the specific consequences such as behavior, emotions, or physical state changes. It is often useful to *incorporate didactic teaching analogies*. For example: "Let's say I spend the night in a friend's large house. I suddenly hear the window pane clank in the neighboring room. If I think: 'Those must be burglars, and I am unarmed and alone,' then I will feel fear. If I think instead: 'It's always the same with me, I must have forgotten to close the window, now the glass pane in the neighboring room is broken,' I will feel anger towards myself." This illustrates to the patient that feelings are not consequences of situations, but rather direct consequences of evaluations of the internal or external situation – an understanding that is essential for patients to recognize. Subsequently, patients are often encouraged to complete records of goal symptom evaluations (such as voice hearing) in the beginning of any cog-

Table 14. Evaluation record: Seeing connections between independent events

Trigger	Automatic thoughts	Alternative thoughts
See red car	• They are trying to tell me something.	• There are many red cars in the world.
	• They are trying to get me to do certain things.	• The color of a car has no bearing on who is sitting in it.
	• They want to control me.	• A car has never harmed me; I am oversensitive.

nitive restructuring. The goal is to work through personal evaluation processes and consequently find a starting point for new evaluations. Table 14 provides an example for the therapeutic processing of dysfunctional evaluations and the establishing of new, more adaptive evaluations.

An additional important strategy is the development of "insight" based on the model of cognitive therapy, when one *makes the clear distinction between experiences and facts*. Misinterpretations can occur at the perceptual level or further along in the processing at the level of event evaluation. The following examples illustrate how we all can and do misinterpret events that happen as part of everyday experiences (Nelson, 1997, p. 94):

1. We hear our neighbors next door having a furious argument but later discover that it was a television program they where watching.
2. We take a walk at night, and the moon in the sky seems to follow us wherever we go. In this case we know that this is an optical illusion.
3. You assume that your friend forgot to send you a birthday card, but later you discover that it was actually sitting at the post office undelivered due to a strike.

Another psychoeducational strategy is to make clear to the patient that *perspectives that were valid in the past are not necessarily true in the present*. Examples for this are the belief in Santa Claus or the feeling of never being able to feel happy again following a breakup with a partner. Also, clinicians might choose to discuss the *difference between experiences and facts*. Useful examples include phantom pain, tinnitus, optical illusions, or day dreams. The important component of these examples is for the patient to learn that *perceptions and reality do not have to agree*.

Conversational psychotherapeutic strategies are also often implemented to change delusional interpretations. The goal is not to mirror the patient's psychotic misperceptions as real. Rather, formulations are used such as "if I were to interpret the situation precisely as you do, then I would also be, e.g., very depressed / very indignant." In other words, clinicians should attempt to capture the patient's interpretive and experience-related frame of reference, and then mirror this perception as understandable in a validating fashion and from an "as if" perspective. This will help stabilize the therapeutic relationship and reduce anxiety and insecurity in the patient. A frequent *problem in the therapeutic relationship results from therapists not agreeing with delusional conclusions*. The following is an example of an intervention for such a scenario that presumably will result in a small burden on the therapeutic relationship (Nelson, 1997, p. 78):

Clear distinction between experiences and facts

Perspectives valid in the past are not necessarily true in the present

Difference between experiences and facts

Perceptions and reality do not have to agree

Conversational psychotherapeutic strategies

Therapists not agreeing with delusional conclusions

I really don't know whether your voices are caused by dust or not; I've never heard of that happening before, but people can react differently to things, so who knows? I agree that the work we've done certainly indicates that the voices are not coming from the people whose voices they appear to be. But I don't suppose it really matters what's causing the voices, the only thing that is really important is to find out what you might be able to do to stop them when they are having a go at you.

A next step can then be to develop hypotheses collaboratively with the patient as to what made him or her receptive to these (delusional) perspectives and psychotic experiences. At this time, one can discuss marijuana use, increase in stress, lack of quality sleep, interpersonal difficulties, life changes such as moves, beginning or end of professional training, even neurobiological factors for developing a psychotic illness. The *important goal is to determine to which "working model" the patient will ultimately commit* and whether this will foster a minimal readiness for cooperation in the patient. The cognitive model – i.e., the powerful effect of evaluation processes on feelings and actions – should be conveyed, as much as a discussion about what triggers "psychotic illness" or "schizophrenic disturbances" in the patient based on possibly incorrect evaluations. In this context, *anti-stigma work should strongly aim to convey the vulnerability–stress–competence model of psychotic disturbances.* Exclusive focus on neurobiological factors alone might potentially motivate greater medication compliance and possibly reduce feelings of guilt. It is, however, not sufficient to promote active coping or willingness for CBT or rehabilitation.

Anti-stigma work

Creating a collaborative *working model about how delusional fears may have developed* is a difficult task. A useful analogy here is that people with psychotic tendencies have a more sensitive *danger detection system* so that feelings of threat appear earlier. Patients then search for an explanation for these feelings, referring to distorted previous learning experiences. Consequently, an explanation is frequently found in the behavior and intentions of others who are present in the situation at hand. A clinical example is a patient who always feels attacked by others if they use the word *um* in his or her presence. In such cases, it is important to work through the following *vicious circle of expectation fear* systematically:

Danger detection system

Vicious circle of expectation fear

Feelings of threat ⇨ hypervigilance ("Um's" mean personal depreciation) ⇨ increase in fear ⇨ additional "sharpening" of perception ⇨ notice more "Um's" ⇨ validation of fear.

The result of this type of vicious circle is the development of expectation fears, which in turn automatically activate feelings of threat in similar future situations.

Clinicians should *not attempt* to completely *remove any potentially existing doubt about such delusional explanations of social situations* but rather engage the patient to collaboratively discuss and recognize that very different explanations and perspectives are possible in social scenarios. Deciding about the appropriateness of these competing interpretations of social situations often depends on how useful they are for guiding behavior in a situation, e.g., to achieve important goals and needs. Specifically, this means encouraging the patient (sometimes despite his or her reluctance) to believe the concept of the vicious circle model. The model will prove itself justified, if the exercise provides an entry point for the reduction of feelings of threat and also provides target items for specific therapy techniques. *Motivating the patient in this way to make new experiences* with new, alternative behaviors (even if initially for a time-limited period), is therefore often an important entry point into changed cognitive evaluations. This can occur in a targeted manner by means of *behavioral experiments* (see below), for which patients are encouraged to check which of several possible alternative explanations is the most helpful.

Motivating the patient

Behavioral experiments

6.2 Strategies for Cognitive Restructuring of Persistent Delusions

A prerequisite for the successful application of cognitive restructuring strategies is that the patient must be motivated to question his or her beliefs and interpretations. The therapist attempts by means of the above-mentioned strategies to motivate patients to generate reasons and counterarguments for the validity of certain conclusions, and to carry out so-called behavioral experiments that have been planned together with the therapist. The latter serve to examine basic assumptions that are associated with the delusional conviction in a goal-directed manner. One needs to consider that patients, due to neurobiologically based changes, are so strongly convinced of their perceptions that they do not seek logical consistency or evidence for the accuracy of these observations. Consequently, the first step often includes *casting of doubt*. This usually succeeds more easily if interventions aim to reduce negative emotional consequences for the patient, e.g., feelings of defeat or fears. *Several cognitive behavioral techniques* are available, such as logical refutation and concrete substantiation.

Casting of doubt

Logical refutation is based on the therapist's question to himself or herself: "Why does it appear implausible or farfetched to accept from the patient that…?" The approach, however, is necessarily tied to the concept of collaborative empiricism: Logical refutation must be emotionally accepted by patients as an instrument with which they can test, with the support of their therapist, whether their perception (e.g., fear) represents the most sensible explanation for a situation or experience. Without collaborative empiricism, the intervention would merely burden the therapeutic relationship and in the worst case lead to treatment termination or even an inclusion of the therapist in the patient's paranoid explanatory model.

Logical refutation

Case Example for the Logical Refutation Method

During the therapy discussion, the patient suddenly becomes anxious or angry. He believes that based on the sound of moving chairs in a room above, people in that room can read his thoughts. The therapist can react in the following manner:

„I see that you are very tense because of the sounds. Would it be helpful if we were to test together [use of the collaborative empiricism principle] if what your emotions are telling you can actually be true? … The room above, just like ours, is located at the rear of the building. So, how would the people in the room above be able to see you come for this session?"

The therapist could continue by carefully signaling a certain sense of surprise and by explaining that the patient's interpretation caused the therapist to be somewhat confused since until now the therapist had always thought that the sounds were caused by chairs being moved on the floor above.

Signaling a certain "surprise"

Signaling a certain "surprise" if the patient makes a delusional statement has the advantage that the therapist indirectly shows, without immediately questioning the credibility of the patient, that not everyone would expect this kind of explanation. Generally, cognitive restructuring must always precede behavioral experiments because patients will not enter into an emotional risk, i.e., to suffer real damage, if they are not convinced that a certain doubting of their views is justified.

Concretely specify delusional content

To concretely specify delusional content is another strategy to introduce doubt. A statement like "someone is following me" is too general to be able to seek confirming or refuting information in present and past situations or to carry out behavioral experiments in a targeted manner. Specifying the delusional content may lead patients to notice that they did not really confront their fears in a differential manner but rather followed their emotions or their intuition.

Avoid confronting the substantially negative emotions

Fear of not being taken seriously

The therapist, however, must always ascertain if inconcrete delusional interpretations and convictions might be due to completely different reasons that could become therapy obstacles unless considered properly. People with delusional symptoms sometimes avoid verbalizing these contents in order to *avoid confronting the substantially negative emotions* associated with them. Patients also often fear substantially negative consequences for themselves and others if they speak about their delusional beliefs: "If I say what I am afraid of, something very bad will happen to my parents!" *Fear of not being taken seriously* or of having to take more medication with a greater risk of side effects could also be a reason for inadequate concrete specification of delusional content. Finally, the *delusional content itself* could be a reason for the patient not to openly address it – e.g., if the patient is deluded into thinking that he is on a secret mission which he may not communicate to anyone. These types of reasons must be precisely clarified before cognitive restructuring is carefully initiated. With every step in the processing of alternative explanations for delusional interpretations, therapists must *determine the patient's flexibility regarding the acceptance of inconsistencies and contradictions,* to avoid burdening the therapeutic relationship prematurely.

Determine the patient's flexibility

Inference chaining

In addition to specifying delusional thought content, *inference chaining* is an important strategy. Cases when a patient's friends or family members previously doubted the patient's delusional thought content or when the same occurs for clinicians usually indicate that something appears inconsistent or contradictory in the argumentation of the patient. These types of inconsistencies and contradictions must initially be clarified: "Why do I believe as a therapist that the patient's fears appear very improbable or implausible?" The response to this question will determine the direction of the therapeutic restructuring process. An example of this intervention is represented in the following case vignette based on Nelson (1997), which clearly illustrates that first all reasons for the patient's conclusions are gathered and verified by the patient: "If it is therefore right that … and also that …, then what your emotions are telling you cannot be right, specifically that …"

For the therapist to decide which inconsistency to work on using inference chaining, it is useful to ask the following question before the intervention: "If this delusional conviction were to be true, what would be the consequences, and what would stand in opposition to the presence?" For example, if a patient believes that a neighbor has magical powers and can predict the future, the therapist could bring up the following question: "Would the neighbor really

---

Case Example for the Use of Inference Chaining

A patient has substantial anxiety since he fears that two caretakers on the inpatient ward will engage in criminal behavior and in that context want to cremate him intentionally. The therapeutic direction of the cognitive work becomes clear as soon as the therapist realizes for himself that such actions not only presuppose antipathy, but also rather substantial feelings of hatred, as well as the willingness to risk being legally responsible for murder and the practicalities of bringing a coffin to the ward, which would then have to be sent to the crematorium and burned there without authorization.

Therapist: If someone likes you, can he also hate you at the same time?

Patient: No.

Therapist: Do you consider both caretakers as rather pleasant or unpleasant when you speak with them?

Patient: Pleasant.

Therapist: Are both of them supportive when you come to them with a problem, or not?

Patient: Supportive.

Therapist: When someone is pleasant and helpful, is this an indication that he likes a person or hates a person?

Patient: That he likes you.

Therapist: You told me that the caretakers are pleasant and helpful to you, so is this an indication that they like you or hate you?

Patient: They like me.

Therapist: Which feelings would a person have when cremating another person while alive? Would he like the other person or hate him?

Patient: Hate him.

Therapist: Do you think that if a person liked another person and did not hate him, that he would then want him to be burned alive?

Patient: No.

Therapist: You know that both caretakers are pleasant when you have contact with them, and they are also helpful when you come to them with problems. You also know that someone who likes you cannot hate you at the same time, but only if someone truly hated you could he want to burn you alive. It therefore appears that both of them do not wish to burn you alive although you sometimes have the feeling that they could want this. What do you think?

---

live in this shabby little rental apartment if he had this talent? He could predict the winning lottery numbers and buy a large house with the winnings." Another example would be to ask a patient with a dermatological hallucination, "If there are really ants crawling under your skin, wouldn't they suffocate due to the lack of oxygen there?" It is important, however, to verify if the patient has or accepts the necessary *factual knowledge* for this type of argumentation, or if it must still be acquired or solidified. For the last example, for instance, it is important to ask if the patient knows that ants need oxygen and knows that there is no oxygen below the skin. Also note, clinicians may certainly introduce new information. It becomes very difficult, however, to destabilize delusional convictions if the patient's revised conclusions must be supported by too much new information. In such cases, the patient can rely on only very little subjectively verified knowledge.

Factual knowledge

Initially, every fact that could be used as counterevidence to delusional convictions later on in therapy must be very well established – cognitively and emotionally. If this is not the case, and *core aspects of the delusional conviction are put into question too early, confirmation bias is likely to occur.* In other words, counterarguments will be reinterpreted to adapt them to the delusional interpretations. Using our earlier example of the patient afraid of being burned alive, the therapist would have to ask the patient repeatedly how he can recognize that both caretakers are friendly toward him. Only then can the therapist contrast this belief with the delusional fear. If the therapist does not assure that the patient truly believes that the caretakers are consistently friendly toward him, the patient will adapt the now questionable counterevidence to the delusional system: e.g., "Yes, perhaps the caretakers did not actually smile at me in a friendly manner, but rather it was a hypocritical grin that should lull me into a feeling of safety."

Solidification of the "pieces of the puzzle"

It is often recommended to separate the *solidification of the "pieces of the puzzle"* (gathering of previous experiences or factual knowledge) and the *putting together of the puzzle* (the logical reasoning) in time. Ideally, this occurs in separate sessions or, if necessary, in the same session but separated by another topic. Consequently, it is very important, to anticipate the possible consequences of the presentation of contradictory evidence to the patient, in order to be well-prepared for the actual cognitive restructuring process.

Keep in Mind: Consider Possible Consequences of Cognitive Interventions!

A subjective (including delusional) conviction is *not* changed if

- it means a decrease in self-esteem
- it reduces the expectation to be able to control one's future and situation
- it increases dislike or
- it increases the feeling of being different from those of the same age and thereby increases the fear of being socially excluded by the peer group

---

Alternative strategies to build and maintain self-esteem, control, pleasure, and a sense of belonging must first be developed if the delusional convictions are maintained by any of these mechanisms. The therapist's approach regarding how to move forward is a decisive factor. He or she must not appear too enthusiastic during the processing of contradictory experiences or appear too assertive when discussing cognitive dissonance between the patient's beliefs and opposing evidence.

Case Example of Inference Chaining (Nelson, 1997, p. 130)

"I've been thinking about what you were telling me last week and something has struck me as a bit strange. You were saying to me that Nurse Smith and Nurse Brown are always pleasant and helpful when they see you or when you ask for something and that that was a good sign that they must like you – and I am sure you are absolutely right in that because people don't do nice things for people if they dislike them. And then I thought about something you were saying the other day that someone would only want to burn someone alive if they really hated them – and that's certainly true. So it occurred to me that as Nurse Smith and Nurse Brown so obviously like you, then they can't hate you, and this would mean that they can't really want to burn you alive after all. Does this make sense? What do you think?"

Even during the successful execution of inference chaining it is important to provide patients with additional emotionally acceptable alternative explanations of how they would reach delusional misperceptions and/or interpretations. An option could be, for example, that they pursued very intense feelings and subsequently resulting automatic thoughts. The separate components of logical reasoning are summarized in Table 15.

Table 15. Steps for logical reasoning

The therapist starts with his or her own impressions

1. Why does the patient's delusional conviction not seem plausible?

2. What potential arguments against the patient's delusional conviction exist, if any?

Detailed analysis of maintaining components for the delusional conviction

3. What experiences and beliefs support the delusional conviction from the patient's perspective?

4. If the patient has existing experiences or beliefs that might contradict the delusional conviction, strengthen them.

5. If the patient has no existing beliefs or experiences, establish appropriate beliefs and knowledge that contradict the delusional conviction.

6. If the patient has inaccurate beliefs or experiences that maintain the delusional conviction, attempt to modify them.

Keep the patient actively involved in cognitive restructuring

7. Anticipate whether there are ways that the patient could resolve for him- or herself any apparent conflict between the delusional conviction and contradicting evidence.

Leave the patient with a clear message

8. Summarize the experiences that contradict the delusional belief. Emphasize why they make sense and what they are based on.

9. Support alternative beliefs that replace the delusion.

(Adapted from Nelson, 1997)

The following is an additional case example to further illustrate the technique (Nelson, 1997).

Case Example for the Use of Logical Reasoning

A patient developed the unpleasant belief that there were little men in his head, based on the sensation of feet pattering from one side of his head to the other. This patient had accepted that he had schizophrenia and knew from earlier therapy that this could produce strange hallucinatory experiences.

Therapist: How do you know the little mean are in your head? How long have they been there?

Patient: I can hear them and feel them running from one ear to the other; they're in a large cavern, I can hear the echoes. They've been there a couple of days, since Sunday night.

Therapist: How many of them are there?

Patient: About half a dozen I think.

Therapist: How big are they?

Patient: About one and a half inches high and half an inch wide.

Therapist: How big is the cavern?

Patient: About seven inches by four inches.

Therapist: How did they get into the cavern?

Patient: Through my ears. They can't have got in anywhere else because, as my friend pointed out, there are no scars on my face.

Therapist: Why do people have heads actually?

Patient: To hold their brains.

Therapist: How big is the brain?

Patient: Almost the same size as your skull.

Therapist: So normally the brain fills the person's head, with no gaps?

Patient: Yes.

Therapist: What does the brain do?

Patient: It sees, hears, and makes you talk.

Therapist: So if someone can see, hear and talk normally does that mean their brain is normal?

Patient: Yes.

Therapist: Can the brain ever get squashed up?

Patient: Yes, if there is a tumor.

Therapist: Does a squashed-up brain work normally?

Patient: No.

Therapist: Would this affect the way the person sees, hears, and talks if his brain was squashed?

Patient: Yes.

Therapist: Can you see, hear, and talk?

Patient: Yes.

Therapist: So if you can see, hear, and talk normally, does that mean you have a normal brain?

Patient: Yes.

Therapist: So if you have a normal brain, that's not squashed up, how can there be a big 7 inch by 4 inch cavern in your head?

Patient: I suppose there can't be.

Therapist: You told me that the little men came through your ears into your head. When I learned biology I was taught that the passage in the ear leads to an eardrum. Did you cover that in your course?

Patient: Yes.

Therapist: What does the ear drum do?

Patient: It vibrates to sounds and this is turned into nerve signals that get sent to the brain.

Therapist: So it can't do this if it is damaged at all?

Patient: No.

Therapist: How do you know the little men did not get in through your face?

Patient: Because they would have left a scar at least half inch across, probably more, so I would have been able to see it.

> **Therapist:** So if they had got in through your ears they would have made a hole at least half an inch across in your eardrum too?
>
> **Patient:** Yes.
>
> **Therapist:** So you would not be able to hear through that ear with a hole that size?
>
> **Patient:** No.
>
> **Therapist:** Can you hear with both ears at the moment?
>
> **Patient:** Yes.
>
> **Therapist:** So you can't have a hole in either of your eardrums, and so the men couldn't have got in that way?
>
> **Patient:** No. I suppose not.
>
> **Therapist:** And you know they can't have got in any other way because there are no scars on your head. And I guess there would have been quite a lot of blood around on your pillow on Monday morning if something as large as one and one half inch by half an inch had forced its way through your skin?
>
> **Patient:** Yes, that's true.
>
> **Therapist:** So, no little men can have gotten into your head? There can't be any little men in your head?
>
> **Patient:** No.
>
> **Therapist:** So it sounds as if the *feelings* you experience of tiny pattering feet running through your head must be another example of your brain hallucinating, but this time through the sense of touch as well as sound. What do you think? It must be a horrible feeling, but I suppose at least it's reassuring to know that there aren't really creatures living in your head and that your brain is still perfectly OK.

6.3 Contradiction and Confirmation of Personal Experiences

Our social knowledge is saved in *scenarios* which represent our social experiences in a generalized form. They are described as cognitive schemas and serve as behavioral guides in our daily social life. Mistrust, such as in paranoid experiences regarding the possibly harmful intent of others, is also represented this way. Experiences conforming to our cognitive schemas are favored for memory and perceptual processes in general and specifically in paranoid experiences, known as *confirmation bias*. Past experiences that are concordant with a patient's delusional explanatory model are more likely to be recalled than contradictory ones. Similarly, perceptual processes "prefer" these types of experiences. Cognitive therapy aims at making these schema-related automatic processes verifiable for the patient. In the case of delusional symptoms, therapists draw both from past experiences and current perceptual distortions, as well as experiences of cognitive work from previous sessions. The central question always targets (subjective) evidence: *"Which experiences confirm the expectations of the patient?"* The therapist systematically prepares the examination of (paranoid) assumptions in behavioral experiments, if necessary together with the patient in session. Many cognitive interventions do not specifically focus on the delusional thought content but rather on the consequences. The cognitive interventions are guided by the thought: "If the patient's (delu-

Central question always targets (subjective) evidence

sional) assumptions were correct what are the associated consequences?" If a patient is convinced that a family member wants to poison him in order to inherit his property, then the therapist would work on the resulting implications with the patient – for example, that the family member would have to show signs of distrust or antipathy, whether the possessions of the patient are even substantial enough for someone to take the risk of possible imprisonment, etc.

Patients do not even seek confirming experiences

Several problems can occur when working on cognitive restructuring of delusional thought content: Some *patients do not even seek confirming experiences*, because the feeling of subjective certainty about their delusional convictions is so strong that any related facts appear completely clear and doubt-free to the patient. In such cases, therapists should react in a *validating manner* with formulations such as "that … is so clear to you that you have never asked what speaks for or against it. Is that right?" To use cognitive techniques in these cases, therapists must first do preparatory work and process with the patient that *feelings of strong certainty can also lead to incorrect assumptions not being questioned.* This should happen without addressing the delusional thought content. A patient will only be able to begin testing his or her subjective assumptions if properly prepared this way. For example, a patient believes that a family member was exchanged with a body double approximately 3 years ago. The patient could ask the questionable double about earlier childhood memories in an attempt to confirm this beliefs. Before the behavioral experiment, however, the therapist needs to precisely determine with the patient what would be correct replies: "What are the responses that a double could not know?"

Occult or esoteric knowledge

Starting points for possible misinterpretations

An additional problem exists if patients refer to *occult or esoteric knowledge* from external sources such as movies or books. In these situations, it can be very helpful for the therapist to become familiar with these ideas by checking the original source to *identify starting points for possible misinterpretations by patients*. For example, a patient might believe that residual symptoms are related to the use of antipsychotic medication, after reading in esoteric literature that psychopharmaceuticals suppress spiritual powers. If the therapist understands the patient's concerns by reading the source literature, he or she can then argue that schizophrenic illness existed before the introduction of antipsychotic medication and also that there are many patients who do not take medications but still suffer from significant impairment.

Distorted thought processes

Another difficulty for cognitive restructuring occurs if the *experiences listed as confirmative evidence* for the accuracy of a delusional conviction *are themselves a result of distorted thought processes*. For example, the delusional conviction "Neighbor X wants to damage my body through electromagnetic waves" can be based on the delusional perception: "I know neighbor X does not like me because of the sly remarks of students that I overheard yesterday in the supermarket." Psychoeducation work regarding perceptual distortions, e.g., personalization, with didactically well-designed examples can sometimes encourage the willingness of patients to examine their conclusions in the therapy setting. If possible, it can be very important and helpful to refer to previously corrected errors in thinking by incorporating them through formulations such as "we found out together that you sometimes have a problem in situations in which events affect you emotionally. In those situations you tend to apply a lot to yourself which at second glance does not have anything to do with you. Could it be possible that you attributed the look of the salesperson as a reference to your presumed ugliness also in this sense?" It is of course important that the therapist does not get lost in details by going after every variation of a delusional topic, but rather addresses core experiences central to dysfunctional assessments and behavior.

One strategy is to *gather contradictory experiences* that challenge delusional interpretations together with the patient. In order not to endanger the therapeutic rapport, therapists should use careful formulations, such as "recently you told me … and you also reported.… If I summarize this for one moment, it slightly confuses me that …" If the therapist then has the impression that the patient does not comprehend an adaptive correction in the delusional conviction, a tactical withdrawal should follow: "Perhaps this is not as important as what I really wanted to speak to you about." It is important that *the delusional concept is precisely defined in a first step.* Let us use the example of a patient who believes that he is "evil to the core." One could work in therapy as follows (Nelson, 1997): "Someone who is evil to the core because he has the devil in him would probably always intend to harm others and would always be happy to see others suffer. This evil person would never do nice things." By taking the patient's concept from a general to a concrete level that can be evaluated, one can then attempt *the second step of gathering counterexamples from the patient's experience.* An appropriate example here would be: "It could be that I am aggressive towards someone, but I am usually sorry about it later on. This would not be the case if I were evil. Then it would make me happy to harm others or to injure others. When I see that others are suffering, I try to comfort them, and I am happy when other people are having fun. In this context, I remember that I recently …"

An additional strategy is the *gathering of confirmatory and also contradictory experiences.* It is important here to avoid forcing premature decisions regarding the accuracy of the delusional convictions. First, the patient is asked to name objectifiable experiences which speak both for and against a delusional argumentation. It is helpful to ask the patient to gather only those experiences that could be used as evidence in a court and thus be verified by a third party. The rationale must always be clear to the patient: That *feelings can be misguiding, including feelings of certainty,* and that the therapist and patient should perhaps systematically verify these experiences together. Throughout the entire process, however, the patient must have the feeling that the therapist only wishes to support the patient in reaching his or her own, if possible, appropriate conclusions. A model that works well is that the therapist keeps a Pro and Con list on which he or she briefly notes the patient's experiences that can then be evaluated in a second step. Prior to evaluating the arguments, however, it is imperative to discuss any confirmatory facts in a critical manner using the Socratic method.

Delusions should be regarded as a type of subjective explanatory model for confusing and anxiety-inducing experiences. Consequently, cognitive restructuring of delusional convictions must always be flanked by the *search for alternative explanations of experiences* that are based on distorted perceptions. *Delusional explanation models should not be "attacked" too early,* because patients could consider the alternative explanation as completely implausible and inapplicable to his or her special circumstances. In the worst case, the therapeutic relationship could be damaged. The patient may experience the

Table 16. Examples of formulations to trigger alternative explanations

- I am asking myself now if it were not also possible that ... or am I completely wrong here?
- Do you believe that there is the possibility that ..., or does this seem completely implausible?
- Based upon what you have just reported, it could also be that ..., but did I even understand you correctly?
- I once knew someone who experienced the same things as you and after a while, he discovered what the actual cause of it was ...
- Do you believe that this could also be a possibility in your case.... Or is this something completely different? I don't know how your family doctor / relative gets the idea that ..., but I would be curious to find out from you on what he bases this?

therapist as disloyal or even include him or her in the delusional system and consider the therapist to be a component in a conspiracy against them. Table 16 lists examples of formulations that aim to carefully stimulate the process of generating alternative explanations in the patient.

Functionality and maintaining conditions

Considerations regarding *functionality and maintaining conditions* of delusional assessments must strategically determine the therapy approach if delusional interpretations are stubbornly maintained because they prevent negative feelings, stabilize self-image and hope, and encourage the expectation of control over the present and future, then alternatives for this function must first be built in therapy. Safety-searching *avoidance behaviors for evading alleged dangers* contribute substantially to the maintenance of delusional beliefs, because contrary experiences are prevented. In these cases, therapists frequently use behavioral experiments (see next section).

Avoidance behaviors

6.4　Reality Testing and Behavior Experiments

Reality testing

Reality testing, the testing of delusional convictions, based on experiences of the patient, should be introduced with a question from the therapist such as "It is difficult for me to determine what could be correct now. However, it could be interesting for us both to take a closer look at the situation. Do you think it would be important for you to find out what is really going on here?" Reality testing refers either directly to the delusional conviction or indirectly to its implications. Below, several examples are given to illustrate the approach of reality testing and behavior experiments. An example in which reality testing refers *directly* to the delusional conviction that a patient is able to read minds is where the therapist suggests for the patient to try reading the therapist's mind in session. The therapist might think of a specific number and write it on a piece of paper, and the patient would then guess the number.

Reality testing can also be *indirectly* applied to implications of delusion. Tests of implications of delusions are usually used if the delusional content is so general or supernatural that it cannot be tested directly: "If that were the case ..., then that would have to ..."

A third example of reality testing and behavioral experiments is seen in patients who think they can influence the thinking of others and are asked to carry out a telepathic experiment. The therapist and patient might agree, for example, that the patient intentionally thinks of provoking a specific situation. The patient goes into a large department store in the direction of a salesclerk and thinks: "There is a fire. You must warn everyone!" Common sense would predict excitement and unrest in the salesclerk if these thoughts truly reached him. Thus, this behavioral experiment would also serve as a reality test for the telepathic capabilities of the patient. If *reality tests* of delusional convictions are very anxiety-inducing for the patient, they should always be carried out in the *presence of a therapist.*

A prerequisite for all forms of reality tests is to discuss the various alternative outcomes of the *behavioral experiment* with the patient ahead of time. Otherwise, the therapist might run the risk that the patient does not challenge the delusional perception but rather gives new meaning to the result of the behavioral experiment. Consequently, the delusional certainty will increase by means of replacement explanations. The following example shows that these types of replacement explanations become more difficult to contradict. A patient who has the delusional conviction that he does not have a brain receives a brain scan as part of a reality test. He then learns by looking at other brain scans how one can recognize the brain on an X-ray before seeing his own scans. Without discussing the possible results of the reality test with the patient in advance, the patient could then explain that the brain he sees in his scanned image is actually not his, but that the radiologist switched the images since he is also part of a conspiracy against the patient. This additional assumption now contributes to a consolidation of the delusional system rather than to its elimination.

Behavioral experiment

An additional example that *insufficiently prepared behavioral experiments may even lead to more difficulties for modifying delusional convictions* is the following: A patient is convinced that as a result of voodoo-like techniques, he can cause a malignant illness in his mother by simply thinking of her. In the context of a behavioral experiment, the patient is asked to concentrate very hard on the health status of his mother, so that her face becomes covered in red pimples. A reality test component of the behavioral experiment was also agreed upon in which the mother was contacted immediately after this experiment, and the patient asked her whether she had developed such a rash. The mother calmed the patient, assuring him that she does not suffer from a rash on her face. Following the experiment, the patient developed the delusional conviction that he had not spoken with his mother, but rather a body double; while the voice sounded similar, the patient believed that it was not exactly her voice. In this case, it would have been better to set up the experiment in a way that the mother could have been brought into session for the patient to see. Should he still have doubts about her being his true parent, he could have asked her questions to which only she would know the answers.

Insufficiently prepared behavioral experiments may even lead to more difficulties

This example shows that behavioral experiments must be prepared very carefully to prevent reinterpretations of contradictory evidence by the patient. If this does happen, the therapist should use *cognitive challenge strategies,* which aim at the "explaining away" of delusion-contradicting information by the patient. The therapist carefully has to offer reasons for why the patient's additional delusional assumptions are implausible. For our example, the therapist might explain that, "There are no body doubles in real life outside of films, and you've dialed your mother's telephone number, so it is unlikely that a possible

Cognitive challenge strategies

body double would have been at her house at that precise point in time. Also, the person on the phone line knew who you were, which would not be the case for a body double. And, the person on the other end of the telephone line was informed of the therapy plan and was consequently not surprised and so it could only have been your mother," etc.

Fluctuating character of delusional symptoms

The possibly *fluctuating character of delusional symptoms can also represent a risk for reality testing and behavioral experiments*, since suddenly changed interpretations or beliefs might make carefully prepared experiments and reality tests obsolete. An example of this might be the patient believing in his telepathic abilities causing harm to his mother, and who might suddenly become convinced that he is being manipulated by electromagnetic waves from Mars. Consequently, the execution of the telepathy experiment does not make any sense because he has now understood that he is actually not provoking a skin rash on his mother's face but rather has to be concerned about his own health and ability to think independently due to being controlled by an outside force. To guard against confusion and to ensure that the therapist has understood the delusional convictions of the patient correctly, the *strategy of paraphrasing* should be used, well-known in client-centered psychotherapy ("Did I understand you correctly that … and therefore …?" "Please correct me if I am wrong, but if I heard you correctly, it sounded like …"). This strengthens the therapeutic connection and avoids misunderstandings as well as context-inappropriate behavioral experiments.

Strategy of paraphrasing

6.5   Long-Term Stabilization of Achieved Therapy Effects

Booster sessions

Following the end of therapy, it certainly makes a lot of sense to carry out *booster sessions* on a continual basis to maintain the effects of therapy. It also helps if patients use *labels* for their psychotic experiences, which can help differentiating them from daily experiences, for example, "I am hearing my voices again." Certain strategies are helpful in cases of a worsening of psychotic symptoms, such as increases or reappearance of voices or delusional thoughts. In cases of recurrence or worsening of illness, delusional thought contents show frequently similar themes. If the patient has previously worked on recognizing which beliefs or which questionable voices require attention and might be indicative of a worsening clinical status, he or she will be able to seek therapeutic assistance earlier, improve, if possible, medication adherence, or apply techniques previously learned in therapy (see Appendices for strategy cards).

7 Why Psychopharmacology May Not Be Enough

This chapter will address common theoretical and clinical management concerns when patients are receiving CBT in parallel with a psychopharmacologic treatment plan. We assume that your clinical orientation is that *antipsychotic medications are indicated for patients with serious mental illness presenting with psychosis.*

Many years ago, research on treatment of psychosis often compared patients who received psychotherapy without antipsychotic medication, with patients who received medication without psychotherapy. One of the prevailing theories at that time was that medication would be counterproductive. Not only was the theory wrong, but it fueled a great deal of antagonism between clinicians who believed in antipsychotic medication and those whose primary treatment modality was therapy. Patients would be caught in the middle of this rift, such that prescribing clinicians often minimized psychotherapeutic approaches and vice versa.

Most of the evidence on efficacy of CBT for psychosis comes from studies in which the behavioral treatment was added to the patient's current medication regimen (see Chapter 3). While it may be somewhat oversimplistic to consider CBT as an "adjunct" to medication, the adjunct analogy is apt when considering how CBT and psychopharmacology might interact. The issue of how a CBT intervention may affect medication adherence will be covered in the next chapter, but there are many other questions and considerations that apply to adherent patients who receive their prescriptions and medication monitoring from one clinician, and enter into a CBT-oriented psychotherapy with another clinician.

7.1 Basics of Using CBT for Patients Treated With Antipsychotic Medication

The starting point is to make sure that the patient, all clinicians, and other stakeholders are aware that *CBT is not meant to be a substitute for antipsychotic medication.* Unlike some other conditions, such as anxiety disorders or depression, for which treatment selection may focus on choosing between CBT and medication, there is no such debate here. Almost all trials of CBT for schizophrenia were done with patients receiving parallel medication management (although often done separately), and *none of these trials attempted to discontinue antipsychotic medication.* Currently, ongoing CBT interventions are being conducted that were designed for patients who do not wish to take antipsychotic medication, but these studies make great efforts to select only those individuals who have already made the decision not to take (or to stop) antipsychotic medication. The secondary question on whether CBT helps maintain medication adherence or, alternatively, somehow encourages nonadherence, will be covered in detail in the next chapter. In brief, CBT is not "against" medication, and most of the currently available books and guidelines for using CBT for patients with psychosis are designed for patients who are being prescribed antipsychotic medication.

With that in mind, the next step is to remember that CBT is not about medication education. Because the key aspect of using a CBT approach is to go with the patient's agenda and not the clinician's agenda, this principle translates into *holding off on medication and disease-based education unless this is specifically requested by the patient.* It is important to remember that violating this rule will change the nature of the therapeutic engagement and would probably mean that the therapy is not really based on CBT principles. This point is emphasized here because it is our experience that the "holding back" on biologically-based illness conceptualization and psychoeducation is probably one of the biggest differences that is immediately apparent; it can be very challenging for clinicians who were trained in psychoeducation to adapt to this difference.

Medications are often insufficient

The premise of using CBT for symptomatic patients taking antipsychotic medications is that *medications are often insufficient for many patients when considering the level of enduring distress and disability* from core schizophrenia symptoms that remain in "stable, medication-responsive" patients. Therefore, we will take a close look at the limitations of antipsychotic medications, which provide the opportunity for better outcomes using a CBT approach. In other words, the overarching philosophy is that CBT can augment antipsychotic medication. These two approaches are meant to complement, not compete with, each other.

However, the often dramatic effectiveness of antipsychotic medications can be deceiving to clinicians and families, who then go on to have unrealistic expectations of the degree to which medications should work, and downplay the downsides and limitations of an exclusive emphasis on this treatment modality. We do not think it is helpful to create a false split between the world of standard pharmacologic treatment and that of the practice of CBT. Doing so would create unnecessary chasms in a field that is already too fragmented.

7.2   A Brief Overview of Antipsychotic Medications

This is a brief overview of antipsychotic medication with an emphasis on the relationship between medication and CBT techniques. For CBT clinicians who also prescribe antipsychotic medications, this is basic but still offers a perspective on integration of CBT and psychopharmacology. This section will review antipsychotic medication, emphasizing those aspects of pharmacologic treatment that directly or indirectly influence the goals and expectations of a course of CBT when added to a medication regimen.

7.2.1 What Are Antipsychotic Medications, and How Are They Classified?

Antipsychotic literally means "against psychosis." Not surprisingly, medications falling into the category of "antipsychotic" have all been shown to reduce or eliminate psychotic symptoms. While these medications often receive regulatory approval for specific psychiatric disorders (e.g., schizophrenia or bipolar disorder), their mechanisms of action are such that they target psychotic symptoms regardless of the underlying cause of psychosis. As will be discussed, this also means that they are not uniquely effective for all of the symptom manifestations of any particular illness or diagnosis.

The terminology used to describe medications that treat psychosis has been the subject of debate and has evolved considerably. In the 1950s, however, the word *antipsychotic* was not commonly used to describe the new medications that had recently become available for the treatment of psychosis and schizophrenia. Between the 1970s and the early 1990s, a much more popular word for *antipsychotic* was *neuroleptic.* Although the words were technically synonymous, psychiatrists mostly spoke and wrote of *neuroleptics* to describe the class of medications available at that time. In fact, *neuroleptic* was the winner of a serious debate among researchers because it deliberately reflected the link between the clinical efficacy of this class of medication and the propensity to cause neurologic effects. This term prevailed because it mirrored the reigning theory at the time that linked the antipsychotic efficacy of these medications with their propensity to cause neurologic reactions, such as parkinsonism, dystonia, akathisia, or dyskinesia. After the advent of the antipsychotic clozapine, this theory had to be abandoned or at least greatly modified. In line with this, the term *neuroleptic* was shelved in favor of the term *antipsychotic.* Even this

Table 17. Antipsychotics approved before and after approval of clozapine*	
Before clozapine **("first-generation" antipsychotics)**	**Clozapine and later developments** **("second-generation" or "atypical" antipsychotics)****
Chlorpromazine (Thorazine, Largactil)	Asenapine (Saphris)
Fluphenazine (Prolixin, Modecate)	Aripiprazole (Abilify)
Haloperidol (Haldol)	Clozapine (Clozaril)
Loxapine (Loxitane)	Iloperidone (Fanapt)
Molindone (Moban)	Lurasidone (Latuda)
Perphenazine (Trilafon)	Olanzapine (Zyprexa)
Thiothixene (Navane)	Paliperidone (Invega)
Thioridazine (Mellaril)	Quetiapine (Seroquel)
Trifluoperazine (Stelazine)	Risperidone (Risperdal)
	Ziprasidone (Geodon, Zeldox)

* Listed alphabetically, not in order of approval (trade names in parentheses).
** These are the antipsychotics approved in the United States since clozapine. Other countries may have other post-clozapine antipsychotics available.

brief review of the history of psychopharmacology of psychosis shows the *importance of giving careful consideration to the naming and classification of these medications*. Naming reflects underlying beliefs of therapeutic targets and mechanism of action, and classification implies the degree to which specific medications share specific features.

7.2.2   What Are the Benefits of Antipsychotic Medications?

Antipsychotic medications are a class of medications that are used to treat psychotic symptoms. As the name implies, these medications are "against psychosis" and not specific to the treatment of schizophrenia. Some of these medications are also used for the treatment of bipolar disorder and persistent symptoms of depression, but we will not address those indications in this book. For persons with schizophrenia or similar conditions such as schizoaffective disorder, *antipsychotic medications are used to help control the acute symptoms of psychosis, and once those are stabilized, also help prevent or delay return of acute symptoms* (relapse prevention). While there have been many studies that have attempted to find ways to discontinue antipsychotic medications, it has been shown that stopping antipsychotic medications will dramatically increase the chances of relapse, and therefore stopping medication is not recommended once the diagnosis of schizophrenia is made. What is often missing in these discussions is that *antipsychotic medications are far from a cure,* in that persons with schizophrenia often continue to have disabling and distressing symptoms even while taking these medications. They also do not address other very common problems of what to do when *a patient does not agree with his or her diagnosis, or does not think medication is needed.* Finally these *medications all have significant side effects*, and clinicians in their efforts to emphasize the benefits often do not fully appreciate the level of distress or discomfort that is connected with having to take these kinds of medications, day in and day out.

7.2.3   What Are the Limitations of Antipsychotic Medication?

Even in the best of circumstances, antipsychotic medications have significant limitations. The most basic limitation that sometimes is forgotten in day-to-day practice is that these medications do not cure mental illness. For someone with a diagnosis of schizophrenia, this means that no matter how well the medication works when the person is taking it, those *benefits will be lost after the medication is stopped.* Often patients will feel better after stopping medication. This is because the *side effects tend to go away faster than the protective effects.* On some level, it is natural for anyone to hope for a cure, and from this perspective medications are disappointing. Aside from this somehow existential disappointment, there are other limitations that are so common that it is easy for practitioners to lose sight of these challenges.

Although antipsychotics are generally most effective for the so-called positive symptoms of schizophrenia, these symptoms often persist despite the best efforts of the patient and prescribing clinician to find the most effective antipsychotic medication regimen. However, the efficacy for positive symptoms, while not ideal, is better than that for many other important symptom domains of schizophrenia. *Antipsychotics are even less likely to be fully effective for negative symptoms* of schizophrenia, and are *relatively ineffective for persistent cognitive symptoms*. Another aspect that should be kept in mind by clinicians reflects the fact that *no medication can reverse the distress, loss, trauma, or stigma that so often accompanies the experience of psychosis*.

Antipsychotics are less likely to be fully effective for negative symptoms and are relatively ineffective for persistent cognitive symptoms

7.2.4   Are There Any Other Limitations in "Real World" Clinical Practice?

In practice, the effectiveness of antipsychotic medication is often compromised by circumstances that further interfere with what may be possible under the best of circumstances. These secondary reasons are often amenable to changes in medication regimen. Other secondary reasons medications fail include the fact that it is not possible to tell in advance which medication will be most effective for any given individual, potentially leading to patients feeling disappointed over limited symptom reduction and possibly reducing their willingness to try a second medication. Also, clinicians may *not prescribe medications in the most effective manner*, and medications may be prescribed at too low a dose, or excessive doses, or too many medications are given such that the patient is overmedicated.

7.2.5   The Problem of Partial Efficacy: Glass Half Full or Half Empty, or Both?

Many prescribing clinicians – and much of the psychopharmacology literature – classify patients as being either a "responder" or a "nonresponder" to prescribed medication. This classification may simplify matters but distorts – and overstates – the effectiveness of medication. Because *antipsychotics are, at best, only partly effective*, it is not realistic to expect that medication will fully control all symptoms of schizophrenia for the vast majority of patients. Therefore, it is more realistic to consider antipsychotic effectiveness on a spectrum of response. Prescribing clinicians should acknowledge that the classification of "responder" and "nonresponder" is somewhat arbitrary and depends on circumstances and expectations rather than any absolute metric. In most clinical settings, the calibration of pharmacologic response is made to the relative response of the patient compared with his or her clinical condition without medication, or roughly calibrated to the expected response in other patients. What often goes unsaid when judging medication efficacy based on the patient's own desire to be well, that is current pharmacologic treatments are almost always inadequate. Unfortunately, clinicians will be seeing medication response from the vantage of how much better the patient is than before, but patients will tend to be keenly aware of the vast chasm between their "optimal" response and how different life remains because of the illness.

Antipsychotics are, at best, only partly effective

7.3 Choosing an Approach: Changing Medication, or a CBT Adjunct?

Table 18. Is a CBT adjunct to medications indicated?

Factor	CBT adjunct indicated	Medications only indicated
Patient motivation	Interest in using a psychological approach for persistent symptoms	Not interested in any psychological treatment approach*
	Unwilling to accept a formal psychiatric diagnosis or biomedical model	Preference for a medication approach to address problem
Medication	Persistent symptoms despite a history of appropriate antipsychotic medication trials	A simple medication adjustment is likely to address concerns
	Switching antipsychotic medication would be considered too great a risk	A primary medication change is a preferred treatment option
	If the next pharmacologic step would be clozapine, the patient is already receiving clozapine or has not done well with or has rejected clozapine	Consider clozapine for patients at very high risk for suicide
	Patient given multiple medications and may have experienced significant side effects or toxicities from medication regimen	Presence of significant adverse effects that can be treated and would otherwise interfere with nonpharmacologic treatments**
Medication adherence pattern	Continued symptoms despite pattern of *good* medication adherence	When *poor* adherence is caused by persistent symptoms rather than intentional decision to discontinue medications
Symptoms	Distress or frustration from positive symptoms that continue despite optimal psychopharmacology	Severe cognitive difficulties or disorganization that limit ability to attend or retain information from CBT sessions
	Any other source of distress or frustration regardless of whether person identifies these as symptoms	Severe paranoid symptoms that are not amenable to initial engagement techniques
		Present symptoms are not causing any distress
Treatment services	Availability of trained clinician in CBT for psychosis	No trained CBT clinicians are available
	Financial and logistical resources available to complete course of CBT once started	Presence of significant opposition or controversy about a CBT approach such that at least minimal consistency across treatment services is not possible

* Often patients have experienced therapies that have emphasized diagnosis or biomedical model, and do not want to continue with that orientation but may be amenable to a CBT approach. The initial evaluation should consider the underlying reason for "lack of interest."

** Examples include significant antipsychotic-induced akathisia such that patient cannot tolerate sessions, significant cognitive problems from anticholinergic medication or from use of multiple medications, severe sedation, etc.

Given the relatively large number of medication options shown in Table 17, prescribing clinicians often change medication in the hopes of finding another medication that is more effective, has fewer side effects, or both. Sometimes this approach is successful, sometimes it is not. While changing medication can be very helpful, it may also mean that there is the risk that a change in medication will lead to a medication that is less effective than the one before (Weiden, 2006; Weiden, Preskorn, Fahnestock, Carpenter, Ross, & Docherty, 2007). Therefore one of the potential benefits of trying a course of CBT instead of changing antipsychotic medication is that it bypasses the risk of changing antipsychotic medication. Table 18 summarizes important factors that should be considered before adding CBT as an adjunct to a patient's medication treatment regimen.

Factors to be considered before adding CBT

8 Cognitive Behavioral Therapy for Psychosis and Medication Adherence

The previous chapter reviewed aspects of medication management and the use of *CBT for individuals whose medications are not fully effective* in controlling distressing symptoms. The assumption in Chapter 7 was, however, that patients are willing and able to take the prescribed medication. Of course, anyone who is familiar with the challenges of treating psychosis is aware that this assumption does not hold for many patients. The current chapter reviews some of the interventions and challenges when considering *CBT approaches for individuals who are at best ambivalent about taking medication* or have already stopped their antipsychotic medication or are likely to do so in the near future.

The chapter addresses the following questions:

(1) Why are patients nonadherent to medication?
(2) Can psychotherapy, like CBT, lead to greater medication nonadherence?
(3) Is CBT safe and effective when given to patients who are not currently taking antipsychotic medication?
(4) Can a CBT approach improve adherence to antipsychotic medication?
(5) How can we adapt CBT to address adherence challenges?

It is very important to remember that a *CBT approach aligns itself with the patient's perspective*, and nowhere is that more of a potential issue than for adherence to medication. Many patients will become skeptical when they catch on to a therapist or clinician whose main agenda seems to be to "sell" antipsychotic medication.

8.1 Understanding Medication Nonadherence: Taking the Patient's Perspective

This chapter will only cover adherence as it pertains to taking recommended antipsychotic medication. The standard definition of medication nonadherence is a "failure or refusal to comply with medication recommendations," and should be familiar to most readers. This definition is a starting point, but not sufficient for understanding the *possible contributions a CBT approach may bring to improving adherence and outcomes.* For example, this definition does not address the efficacy of the prescribed medication, such that strictly speaking, nonadherence is linked to disobedience to the prescribing clinicians rather than effectiveness of the prescribed medication. The definition also does not define the extent of the difference between what is prescribed and what is taken, in order to meet criteria for nonadherence. *Very few people do exactly as their doctor tells them,* and calling any medication deviation "nonadherence" would trivialize the concept (Velligan et al., 2006b). Taken together, the definition of medication nonadherence does not inform clinicians or patients about the extent to which "failure or refusal to comply with medication recommendations" contributes to poor outcome. Finally, the standard definition docs not cover the full range of attitudes that ultimately determine whether the medication regimen is taken as prescribed. Therefore, in clinical practice it is helpful to consider adherence attitudes as well as adherence behaviors (Velligan et al., 2009b; P. Weiden, 2007).

As a prelude to the treatment implications for the CBT-oriented clinician, let's review some of these adherence issues and how they might apply to the therapeutic intervention.

- Because the standard definition of *nonadherence* involves "failure or refusal" to follow a recommendation, it has the potential to threaten the therapeutic relationship. A CBT approach needs to *address adherence in a way that strengthens rather than erodes the therapeutic relationship.*
- Adherence is a means to an end, in that it must become apparent to the patient why *medication adherence can ultimately be of benefit.*
- There are many reasons any possible benefits of medication will not be apparent to the patient even if it is apparent to others. These include the problem of partial efficacy discussed in Chapter 7, the lag time between starting medication and therapeutic response, as well as the lag time between discontinuation and worsening of symptoms, associations of taking medication with the stigma of having a mental illness, and interference with reaching life goals.
- For any adherence intervention to be effective, the therapeutic relationship must be established, the patient's beliefs and understanding of medication has to be understood, and only then can there be an attempt to review the role of medication in achieving the goals established in the CBT problem list.

Just as Chapter 7 highlighted the importance of the limitations of antipsychotic medication as a way to understand the potential rationale for using CBT interventions, it is important for the CBT clinician to understand the benefits of antipsychotic medication before addressing adherence issues. Please keep in mind that because you, the reader, understand these benefits does not mean that patients will automatically agree or even accept these perspectives. In fact, perhaps one of the reasons that psychoeducation alone does not improve adherence is that these kinds of facts are presented without *consideration of the readiness of the patient to listen or understand.*

8.1.1   Impact of Adherence Problems on Clinical Outcomes

Relapse go up almost fourfold

Clinicians reading this textbook are probably aware that nonadherence can have terrible consequences on outcomes. The time-adjusted chances of *relapse go up almost fourfold after an acute psychotic episode for patients who stop their medication* compared with those who stay on their medication (chances of relapse are 11% per month for non-adherent patients compared with 3% per month for adherent patients). Those relapses associated with nonadherence tend to be more likely to lead to permanent harm, such as suicide, accidental death, or arrest (Leucht & Heres, 2006).

Until recently, there was more debate whether so-called partial compliance, defined as taking less but some of the prescribed antipsychotic, is detrimental to long-term outcome. In theory, perhaps the dose–response characteristics of antipsychotics are such that many patients could take some but not all of their medication without suffering any adverse consequences. In fact, many clinicians believe that antipsychotics are "forgiving," and brief medication gaps (e.g., over weekends) do not adversely affect therapeutic outcome. However, there is a significant sensitivity to the extent to which there is partial compliance and subsequent relapse. Using pharmacy refills as a proxy for medication gaps, nonadherence was associated with poorer functional outcomes. A study using pharmacy refill data in a primarily adherent cohort chosen to be at low risk for relapse showed that *medication gaps of up to 10 days can double the odds of hospitalization* (Weiden, Kozma, Grogg, & Locklear, 2004). In clinical practice, there are significant consequences, such as increases in symptoms and relapse, even for patients who are partially non-adherent, and those patients seem to be more impaired and relapse more often than patients who take antipsychotic medications regularly as prescribed.

Medication gaps of up to 10 days can double the odds of hospitalization

There are other ways in which adherence issues can jeopardize therapeutic outcomes. Some of these ways are indirect, by obscuring the pharmacologic response to medication, eliciting medication decisions that can be harmful, and jeopardizing the clinician–patient relationship. In day-to-day practice it can be difficult to disentangle the causes of relapse attributed to nonadherence from loss of efficacy for other reasons. These indirect effects – harm to the therapeutic alliance, reducing the apparent effectiveness of medications – are amenable to some of the CBT techniques described in greater detail later in this chapter.

Table 19. Key points on medication adherence

- Nonadherence is very common in any persistent illness, and many reasons that mentally ill patients stop medication are no different from those for other conditions.

- Adherence and nonadherence can change over time, such that individuals who are adherent at one time may stop medication at another time.

- In clinical practice it is very difficult to accurately assess medication adherence. Clinicians often miss the degree or extent to which nonadherence occurs in their own practice.

- Adherence is usually considered as a behavior (take/not take medication), but it is also an attitude (want to take/opposed to taking medication).

- Sometimes, nonadherence is caused by practical difficulties taking medication regularly, and sometimes it is based on an active decision.

For the purposes of CBT interventions, two other challenges need to be considered. First, it is very *difficult to accurately assess adherence status*. Prescribing clinicians tend to underestimate nonadherence – in other words, they believe that their patients are adherent when in fact many are really non-adherent but do not disclose this to their clinicians. Many patients cannot or will not fully disclose the actual extent to which they are missing medication. Another problem is that many clinicians are not aware of *the extent to which nonadherence goes on undetected!* The true nature of the nonadherence problem is often revealed after the patient has a relapse or a crisis. Key points on medication adherence are summarized in Table 19.

Accurately assess adherence status

8.1.2   The Importance of Understanding Adherence Attitudes

The standard definition of nonadherence focuses on adherence behavior more than adherence attitudes. In other words, nonadherence is defined by what the patient does with medication (take or not take), and is less concerned about why the patient was non-adherent. For patients with psychosis, sometimes the nonadherence comes out of an *intentional decision to stop medication* ("I don't need the medication anymore," or "I have a new sexual partner and the medication causes sexual difficulties"). But often the nonadherence is related to some other factor that is an obstacle to adherence, where under other circumstances the patient would be perfectly willing to continue with medication (e.g., the patient is too symptomatic or forgetful to go to the pharmacy to pick up medication, or the patient uses street drugs and is too "high" to remember to take medication). It is very important to know whether the patient wants to take medication, wants to stop, or has ambivalent attitudes about adherence.

Intentional decision to stop medication

At any given moment, patients may have one or more reasons for taking medication, and simultaneously have others that influence them toward nonadherence. All of these attitudes can coexist and can also fluctuate based on circumstances such as changes in symptomatology or social environment (Ajzen, 2001). *Attitudinal shifts do not always match clinical effects.* For example, a patient who believes medication is helpful because it lessens the intensity of voices may conclude that medication is no longer necessary, after changing to another medication that completely eradicates those voices. Attitudes also frequently shift when there are *changes in social relationships* with subsequent changes in social influence. For example, a patient is likely to be more distressed by medication-induced sexual difficulties when starting a new relationship. The presence of competing attitudes, some favorable and others unfavorable, is sometimes described as *attitudinal ambivalence* (Conner, Povey, Sparks, James, & Shepherd, 2003). This term reflects the person's holding *coexisting positive and negative dispositions toward the attitudinal object* – in this instance, the idea of taking or continuing with psychiatric medication. For example, a patient may say that he or she remains adherent because "it helps calm me down and I would get upset without it," yet also report that "I want to stop my medication because it does not work for me; I'm still feeling suicidal and hearing voices"!

Attitudinal shifts do not always match clinical effects

Coexisting positive and negative dispositions

The reader may have already guessed that a CBT approach is very well suited for assessing and understanding adherence attitudes. In many ways, the overall approach taken for adherence issues will be no different from that for other core problems that are being driven by symptoms that are not immediately apparent to the patient. We will revisit this in greater detail at the end of this chapter.

8.2 Can a CBT Approach Encourage Nonadherence?

Because a CBT approach does not intuitively align with a biomedical model of schizophrenia, there is a concern that a CBT-oriented psychotherapy might be interpreted as rejection of a pharmacologic treatment model. Indeed, there is a historical basis for this concern. In the previous era of psychoanalytically oriented psychotherapy, often there would be a direct conflict between the therapist and the prescribing clinician. In those days, sometimes antipsychotic medications were considered contraindicated because they would "mask" the

CBT approach is not "against" medication

symptoms and interfere with therapy. The important point here is that a *CBT approach is not "against" medication, by any means.* Furthermore, patients are not encouraged to discontinue medication. Most frequently, CBT is offered as an adjunct treatment option in addition to antipsychotic medication.

A historical case example illustrating the tension between pharmacologic and psychoanalytically oriented therapy is depicted in the biography of John Nash, a brilliant mathematician who developed schizophrenia in the early 1960s. In *A Beautiful Mind,* the biographer Sylvia Nasar describes how theories of schizophrenia were conveyed to patients during that era (Nasar, 1998). The onset of Nash's schizophrenia in the late 1950s coincided with the recent introduction of chlorpromazine (the first modern antipsychotic). When Nash was initially diagnosed with schizophrenia, medications were not accepted as a mainstream treatment for schizophrenia. "Nobody thought of Thorazine as anything but an initial aid in preparing the way for psychotherapy" (p. 259). Put into today's language, Nash's "psychoeducation" would consist of his illness being described as caused by "fetus envy" because his presentation coincided with his wife's pregnancy, and he would be informed that psychotherapy was absolutely essential and that antipsychotic medication was a second-class treatment. After this experience, Nash only accepted medication under duress, and would quickly stop medications despite the clear evidence that they were effective for his psychosis. While there may have been many reasons for his persistent nonadherence, his *initial experience with psychiatric treatment clearly led to a skeptical if not refusing attitude toward medication.*

No evidence that a CBT approach increases nonadherence

Despite reasonable concerns, there is *no evidence that a CBT approach increases the likelihood of nonadherence.* In fact, the opposite is presumably true. There is more evidence that a strictly biomedical model educational approach does not seem to improve medication adherence. Anecdotal evidence suggests that in fact such an approach may backfire for some individuals who recoil at the diagnosis of schizophrenia, or cannot tolerate the idea of accepting a diagnosis of severe mental illness, and link the recommendation of medication with acceptance of such a diagnosis. For those individuals, a CBT approach may actually improve adherence by bypassing such a biomedical model and allowing a more acceptable model of medications as being part of a treatment plan

Table 20. Key points about whether CBT can trigger medication nonadherence

- The historical background for this concern is that around the time antipsychotic medications were introduced, psychoanalytically oriented psychotherapy was also a treatment for psychosis. In that era, many of the therapists would be openly opposed to antipsychotic medication.
- Current CBT approaches are not opposed to antipsychotic treatment and do not communicate "antimedication" beliefs.
- Biomedical model psychoeducation is not very effective for promoting or sustaining medication adherence; therefore patients are likely to be more adherent when CBT is used instead of biomedical model psychoeducation.
- Research comparing CBT with other therapies or with treatment as usual, does not show any sign of greater nonadherence in groups assigned to CBT. Some small studies show improvements in medication adherence associated with a CBT intervention.
- Based on the patient-centered literature, adherence interventions that stay congruent with the persons' inherent health beliefs are more likely to improve adherence than more "generic" educational approaches.

that fits better into the patient's own self-understanding of his or her condition (see Table 20).

One may ask whether there is a tacit or implicit antimedication message if a patient embarks on a psychotherapy that does not necessarily endorse a biomedical model of schizophrenia or psychosis. In other words, for those patients who reject a medical model, *a CBT approach will not try to "educate" the patient into a forced view* of his or her condition as being biologically based. One could argue that this may give permission for patients to stop their medication, whereas otherwise they would have remained on medication using a more traditional psychoeducation approach. Remember that the essential component of a CBT approach is to *establish a working alliance using*, as much as possible, *the person's own concept* of the nature of the problem. In this way, a CBT therapist would not challenge a patient's own explanation of what is wrong, including those who already are, or prefer, viewing their condition from a biomedical model perspective and those who do not. The essential philosophy here is not so much that CBT opposes a biomedical model, rather that it does not force it on those who are "turned off" by it. It seems that *many patients are perfectly able to work with two different treatment approaches*, as long as these approaches do not directly contradict each other.

Establish a working alliance

8.3   Is CBT Appropriate for Patients Who Refuse Medication?

This is an area of some debate. Let's start by reviewing what is known. The concern about using CBT and other active psychotherapies is based on earlier research that some kinds of psychosocial therapies that are helpful for patients taking medication can be counterproductive for patients who are off medication. The classic study showing such an effect was done in the 1970s (Hogarty, Goldberg, & Schooler, 1974), when it was still considered ethical to randomize outpatients with schizophrenia to medication and no-medication conditions. In this study, recently discharged outpatients with schizophrenia were randomized to one of four groups in a 2 × 2 design. Half of the subjects received a rehabilitation therapy called major role therapy (MRT), and half did not get any therapy. Half received antipsychotic medication (chlorpromazine), and half received placebo. The group who received BOTH active medications AND MRT did best. This was no surprise. But what was surprising to the researchers was that among the group of patients who did not receive any medications, those receiving MRT were more likely to relapse than those who were not in any active psychosocial therapy.

While surprising at the time, the benefit of hindsight provides a sensible explanation for this finding. The goals of MRT were rehabilitation and reintegration, which can be very stressful and grueling for many patients who have recently relapsed and are trying to contend with their symptoms as well as get back to day-to-day functioning. Presumably being in MRT was more stressful than not being in MRT. Patients who were taking antipsychotic medication were more likely to benefit from MRT because medication was helpful in providing a cushion or buffer to help mitigate the impact of stress. Without antipsychotic medication, however, MRT was more likely to cause more stress than the patient could handle at the time. The lesson here is that the *stress of the therapy probably triggered breakthrough psychosis in patients* who were not taking medication, whereas those who were on medication were resilient enough to handle the challenges of therapy. The results of this study, and some others like it, were very influential. The lesson was to hold back on offering any goal-oriented psychosocial or psychotherapeutic intervention for patients who were not currently taking antipsychotic medication.

With this background, it would not be surprising to assume that a CBT-oriented psychotherapy might increase psychotic symptoms or relapse for patients who are not currently taking medication. Fortunately this does not seem to be the case. The recent evidence for *CBT differs in that there is no apparent harmful effect of this approach for patients who are not currently taking antipsychotic medication* (see Chapter 3). Therefore, while *CBT is not a substitute for antipsychotic medication*, it does not seem to be harmful, and some preliminary studies suggest that it may even be helpful for some symptoms (Table 21).

Stress of therapy probably triggered breakthrough psychosis

Table 21. Key points about starting or continuing CBT for patients who are not taking antipsychotic medication
• CBT has been shown to be helpful in patients who were at high risk for converting to psychosis and are not yet on medication.
• One pilot study of CBT in "first-episode" psychosis patients who choose to stay off medication shows some symptom improvement despite absence of medication.
• In the "real world," CBT may already be given to patients who are not taking antipsychotic medication, if the CBT clinician is simply not aware of the change in medication status.
• Any intervention that helps maintain the therapeutic alliance after medication cessation will lower the risk of hospitalization or other problematic outcomes.
• Although not yet proven for CBT, interventions that improve the therapeutic alliance in schizophrenia are likely to be useful.

Table 22. Key points about whether CBT techniques may be used as a means to improve adherence

- Maintaining the therapeutic relationship is always a primary objective, and great care should be taken to discuss adherence issues in a way that does not alienate the patient.
- *Assess adherence behavior but do so in a way that is nonjudgmental and nonconfrontational.* If you learn of nonadherence, try not to "lecture" or "scold" the patient.
- Assessing patients' adherence attitudes is most important for developing a better understanding of beliefs and attitudes about adherence. Use guided discovery techniques to clarify vague or inconsistent statements about adherence. Make sure that you *understand all major reasons from the patients' perspective*, and avoid making "corrective" statements too soon.
- Use standard CBT techniques such as normalizing nonadherence and patient's reasons for rejecting medication, especially on issues such as stigma, disagreement over biomedical model, and frustration over partial efficacy of medications.
- Suggestions about adherence are best introduced after the full adherence assessment is completed and brought into the shared goals already established by the problem list.
- Do not be critical or judgmental when patients stop their medication, rather use a "harm reduction" approach, and *maintain the therapeutic relationship despite nonadherence.*

Nonjudgmental and nonconfrontational

Maintain the therapeutic relationship despite nonadherence

Despite the importance of the problem, there is very *little prospective research* on whether using a CBT approach can improve adherence or prevent subsequent nonadherence. Most of the efficacy studies of CBT aimed to reduce persistent symptoms among schizophrenia patients who are thought to be adherent to their antipsychotic medication. Some of the meta-analyses also found *lower dropout rates for patients assigned to CBT* compared with those on treatment as usual. Specifically, patients assigned to CBT interventions were more than twice as likely to remain in treatment compared with control patients (pooled odds ratio = 0.38). Although dropout from therapy is not the same as medication nonadherence, this finding supports the hypothesis that CBT may be better than other approaches in engaging patients in a therapeutic relationship (Table 22).

Lower dropout rates for patients assigned to CBT

Why might a CBT approach be helpful for improving medication adherence for patients with schizophrenia? Because CBT focuses on beliefs and attitudes, it may be helpful for patients who actively decide to discontinue their medications, a situation that frequently occurs with schizophrenia patients. A *CBT approach would not be expected to be useful when nonadherence is unintentional*, perhaps related to persistent cognitive or negative symptoms that are major barriers to adherence. For those individuals, it is not their attitude that leads to nonadherence, but rather their illness that interferes with their ability to stay adherent with medication.

CBT approach probably not useful when nonadherence is unintentional

8.4 Using CBT to Assess and Improve Adherence

As mentioned, many of the core techniques used in the practice of CBT for psychotic disorders can be applied to the issue of adherence. What changes is the focus of CBT rather than the way CBT is used. Many patients have significant problems with maintaining reasonable medication adherence over time. There are many underlying reasons for nonadherence that become very relevant in deciding whether a CBT-oriented intervention would help. With that in mind, this section covers some of the steps to consider when addressing adherence and related challenges.

8.4.1 Frame Any Adherence Discussion in a Way That Preserves the Therapeutic Alliance

CBT clinician has to balance his or her role with the prescribing clinician

Adherence is a behavior that depends on at least two people – the prescriber and the patient. Adherence, then, can reflect relationship issues between the prescriber and patient. Inasmuch as the therapeutic alliance is fundamentally essential for all aspects of treatment of schizophrenia, it is important to do everything one can to preserve or enhance the therapeutic alliance. When CBT is done by a nonprescribing clinician, as is often the case, the *CBT clinician has to balance his or her role with the prescribing clinician.* When conflict or power struggles exist between the patient and prescribing clinician or treatment team, it is important to try to *avoid taking sides.* It is not consistent with a CBT approach to try to talk the patient into being adherent with medication. Likewise, overselling of medication benefits or excessive enthusiasm about the importance of medication is likely to backfire and possibly hurt the alliance.

Nonadherence as an "experiment" with certain "learning points"

Another aspect of the therapeutic alliance is to avoid "burning bridges" during instances when the patient stops medication or drops out of treatment. Using *fear communication* such as saying "I know you are going to relapse" can be counterproductive (Leventhal & Watts, 1966). It is better to view these occasions as being a part of the natural course of illness, and maintain a stance of persistence over time despite nonadherence. Clinicians should take a *harm reduction* approach such that even if relapse occurs, the preservation of the therapeutic alliance will hopefully allow the person to reenter treatment earlier. Finally, in the aftermath of a relapse that was triggered by nonadherence, it is best to avoid an "I told you so" kind of attitude which will be viewed as patronizing. It is much better to do a "debriefing" and consider what the lessons learned are. One way to normalize this process is to describe the *nonadherence as an "experiment" with certain "learning points."*

8.4.2 Make Sure That You Assess Both Adherence Attitude and Adherence Behavior

Concerns about the clinician's reaction

Behavior and attitude, while related, need to be considered separately. Most of the adherence assessments go as far as asking whether or not the patient took medication regularly between visits. That is asking about adherence behavior. It is even more important in a CBT context to ask about adherence attitudes. While patients may *not be entirely forthcoming about their adherence behavior because of concerns about the clinician's reaction,* it is our experience that they are more willing to share medication beliefs and attitudes because disclosing those is not necessarily linked to the socially undesirable result of medication nonadherence. Furthermore, a CBT approach is more amenable to working with attitudes and beliefs, and helping guide and correct dysfunctional beliefs. Therefore, assessing and understanding the full range of adherence attitudes is the first step in a CBT-oriented adherence intervention.

8.4.3 Understand the Full Spectrum of Adherence Influences Before Commenting on Adherence

It is very important to hold off on comments or suggestions on adherence information until the entire adherence assessment is finished. To illustrate the importance of this, let's consider an ordinary social situation when asking for advice from a friend. Assume you are struggling with a difficult decision. You call a friend for help and advice. You start to tell your friend about the situation. Before you have finished telling your story, your friend starts to tell you what you should do. Many people feel frustrated when they get advice before they have had the chance to tell their entire story. Even if the advice is perfectly solid and based on adequate information, chances are good that the person getting the advice will not feel heard or understood.

8.4.4 Normalize Nonadherence and Nondisclosure of Nonadherence

Normalizing is a basic yet very powerful CBT technique. Because much of the time, patients feel like being non-adherent is "bad" or that honest reporting of nonadherence would lead to disapproval or worse, *normalizing can be very useful during any part of an adherence assessment or intervention.* Patients are often anxious or defensive when a clinician brings up adherence, and normalizing can be very effective in reducing this tension.

Normalize nonadherence and nondisclosure

8.4.5 Frame Any Discussion of Adherence Problems in Terms of Desired Outcomes, Not Obedience

If and when it is time to bring up a discussion of medication adherence to address specific adherence problems, the dialogue should always start with a review of shared outcome goals. Clinicians may assume that the connection between adherence and outcome is understood, but the understanding is often not shared by the patient, or may be shared in a way that differs substantially from your own (Heinssen, 2002). Because of the power imbalance in many therapeutic relationships, patients often expect that any adherence discussion will be an admonishment, or that the clinician will be angry with them for partial or nonadherence. This should be kept in mind whenever addressing this issue. One approach is to *always start with the desired treatment goals that are shared between the patient and clinician.* There will not always be agreement on how to reach those goals, but this will frame the adherence discussion as being part of the clinician's desire to achieve a shared goal rather than arising out of a desire to control or elicit obedience. As much as you can, try to *keep the discussion about medication adherence positive* – even enjoyable. Above all, try to maintain and even strengthen the alliance, even if there is disagreement about the need for medication.

Always start with the desired treatment goals

Keep discussion about medication adherence positive

Table 23. Some guided exploratory questions about medication attitudes and experiences

Medication experiences and expectations

- Past experiences with medication: Were they good? Bad?
- Current perception of medication effects: Do meds help with anything? Make anything worse?
- Expectations of what staying on medication would do in the future

Burden of taking medication

- What hardships are imposed by medication?
- Are there any hassles or difficulties with the medication regimen, such as paying, figuring out how to take it, etc?
- Are there any side effects that cause distress or discomfort?
- Do any side effects interfere with relationships?
- Do any side effects interfere with future goals?

Usefulness of taking medication

- Does medication make life easier in any way?
- Does medication help deal with stresses or day-to-day problems?
- Do medications help with relationships?
- Do medications help you feel better in any way?

Medications and your prescribing clinician

- Why does your clinician want you to take medication?
- Do you worry that your prescribing clinician has any hidden reasons for recommending medication that are not explained to you?
- Is your prescribing clinician worried about the side effects of the medication?
- Does your clinician do anything that makes it easier for you to stay with medication?
- Does your clinician do anything that "turns you off" to the idea of taking medication?

Opinions of others about your taking medication

- Do other people know about your taking medication?
- Does anyone have any opinions on that?
- Who do you go to for advice on medication?
- Who wants you to take medication?
- Who wants you to stop taking medication?
- What happens when someone's opinion about medication is different from yours? Does this cause any stress or difficulties for you?

Your opinion about yourself when taking medication

- Do you feel embarrassed or ashamed to take medication?
- Do you feel like taking medication is a step toward staying healthy?
- Do you think taking medication is a sign of weakness?
- Does medication help you feel good about yourself?

8.4.6　Eliciting Medication Attitudes and Experience

Because adherence problems frequently aggravate many of the goals set up in the problem list, it is often appropriate to do a focused adherence assessment. In our experience, it is unlikely for most patients that they have ever had an in-depth assessment in a relaxed, collaborative manner where tensions associated with obedience and power issues are put aside. In general, if the CBT clinician is not also the prescribing clinician, it is likely that medication and medication adherence is not going to appear directly on the initial problem list. We have found that the *adherence assessment interview is best done shortly after the problem list is generated*, such that adherence attitudes can be incorporated into the larger therapeutic plan of action. The CBT clinician, in collaboration with the patient, needs to decide ahead of time *whether or not confidential information about nonadherence will be shared with the prescribing clinician*. We suggest that if possible *the responses on adherence should be kept confidential*, especially early on, to foster honest dialogue and safety in disclosure. However, this recommendation may not be consistent with internal treatment policies, and the policy should always be clarified prior to doing a formal adherence assessment as part of a CBT intervention. Then, the policy should be shared with the patient prior to commencing the formal adherence assessment suggested here. It can also be helpful for the nonprescribing CBT clinician to clarify his or her relationship with the prescribing clinician, as well as their lines of communication, so there are no confidentiality misunderstandings later on. Again, the principle in play here is to make sure that *whatever happens in the adherence assessment will not compromise the therapeutic alliance*.

Responses on adherence should be kept confidential

Table 23 illustrates some types of interview questions that can help with the adherence assessment. While it may not be realistic to ask all of these specific questions, they serve as a guide for the type of gentle exploration that can be part of the adherence attitude assessment. In general, a starting point is wherever the clinician feels the topic is most aligned with the specific interests and issues of the patient. What is not shown in text, but is equally important, is the tone in which the discussion takes place. It is very *important to convey curiosity in a nonjudgmental fashion*. Above all, it is crucial during this exploratory phase to *avoid contradicting or correcting what is said by the patient*. Obtaining information and understanding is your goal. Any intervention can come later.

Convey curiosity in a nonjudgmental fashion and avoid contradicting or correcting what is said by the patient

8.5　Indications for the CBT Adherence Intervention

Once there is an understanding of adherence issues and challenges facing the patient, then the clinician needs to decide whether a CBT-oriented adherence intervention might be useful. Why would CBT be useful for preventing medication nonadherence for persons with schizophrenia? Since CBT focuses on changing attitudes, it may be ideally suited for addressing adherence problems in patients who do not believe they are ill. Patients who do not think they have schizophrenia will not be receptive to an adherence strategy that presupposes acknowledgment of having such an illness. A theoretical advantage of a CBT approach for schizophrenia treatment is that it may be acceptable to those individuals who cannot or will not accept a diagnostic label. Thus, a CBT-based adherence intervention might be able to *bypass the tension inherent in having to acknowledge having a mental illness* (Turkington, Kingdon, & Weiden, 2006b; Weiden et al., 2006b).

The potential strengths of a CBT approach for improving adherence in face of negative attitudes to medication can point to when other adherence interventions might be more suitable. There are other common causes of adherence problems where a CBT-oriented intervention would probably not be indicated or, even if adherence is a problem, would be unlikely to be helpful. Because there are so many reasons behind adherence difficulties, it is important to best match the reason with an intervention that is most amenable to addressing the specific problem. To give some extreme examples, a CBT intervention will not help someone who is too symptomatic to attend sessions or too disorganized to take medication without assistance. Rather, increasing the level of supervision, or finding a more effective medication, would be reasonable choices in those patients. Alternatively, increasing the level of supervision is not going to be helpful for someone who rejects medication because of stigma. Table 24 offers some suggestions for situations in which a CBT adherence intervention might

Table 24. Is a CBT adherence intervention indicated?

Primary adherence issue	CBT adherence intervention approach	Other adherence approaches
Patient is not accepting medication, because of acute psychotic symptoms	Not indicated as primary intervention	Reassurance, safety assessment, structured environment such as inpatient unit
Patient is unable to take medication, because of symptoms affecting adherence behavior, such as disorganization	Not likely to address symptom barriers	Consider behavioral interventions to help structure medication taking or long-acting injections for monitoring
Family member or someone influential opposed to medication	No, not a primary approach, unless it includes family	Family psychoeducation
Patient is only willing to accept treatment if clinician uses nontraditional model of illness	Yes, is a primary approach	Biomedical model psychoeducation may inadvertently aggravate adherence problem
Patient is unwilling to take medication, because of "denial of illness" or "lack of insight"	Yes, is a primary approach	Biomedical model psychoeducation may inadvertently aggravate adherence problem
Patient is ambivalent about medications for unknown reason	Yes, to help understand adherence issues from patient-centered perspective	Other interventions may help

be most helpful, and also when other types of interventions might be more appropriate.

8.6 Understanding Adherence Attitudes: The Health Belief Dialogue

The health belief dialogue (HBD) was developed to facilitate a medication adherence intervention based on CBT principles (see Table 25). Assuming the CBT therapist decides to tackle negative or possibly distorted concerns about medication, the *HBD is used to guide the patient and therapist into generating a shared list of reasons that review the advantages and disadvantages of medication from the patient's point of view*. This list can be reviewed and made part of the CBT process, such as in guided questions or behavioral experiments. Once established, the goal is to bring about attitudinal changes based on the patient's own inherent beliefs and motivations rather than "one size fits all" educational messages about the role of medication.

Having conducted many HBD interviews, we find that certain themes come up repeatedly, some of which are covered in the following sections.

Review the advantages and disadvantages of medication from the patient's point of view

8.6.1 Addressing "Lack of Insight"

One of the most common challenges in maintaining ongoing medication adherence is the degree to which patients with schizophrenia do not acknowledge having an illness or needing treatment in the first place. CBT could promote adherence in such patients who feel stigmatized by the diagnostic label of schizophrenia. CBT advocates and promotes personal disclosure and provides a comfortable therapeutic environment by *normalizing challenging disclosure content,* including nonadherence to medication. Even in patients with partial or full insight, adherence is often poor due to a variety of concerns, such as that medications will have sedative effects, making the patient unable to fight off persecutors or antagonistic voices. In such cases, education about paranoia would be counterproductive, whereas acceptance of the patient's point of view might be better able to facilitate an adherence "compromise" resulting in some medication acceptance. Such partial compliance, e.g., at subtherapeutic doses, would certainly not be considered effective medication treatment. The purpose here would be to keep the patient actively involved in the medication dialogue and some medication adherence routine, with the goal to eventually reach therapeutically effective doses.

Normalizing challenging disclosure content

A CBT approach can also provide a model for how psychotic symptom experiences are maintained, which can include an explanation of the need for stress reduction and sleep, which antipsychotic medication can provide and which aid effective coping.

Similarly there are many core personal beliefs which can wreck adherence (e.g., "I can't succeed if I'm on medicines"; "Medications are a sign of weakness"; "Being on medication proves that I am a damaged person"). These personal beliefs can be worked with during adherence sessions, leading to the

Table 25. Adherence Attitude Interview Worksheet

Advantages	Adherence Influence	Disadvantages	Adherence Influence
Patient believes there is an illness that needs to be treated with medication	☐	Patient does not agree that there is an illness or condition in need of medication	☐
Taking medication achieves some day-to-day benefits	☐	No benefits associated with taking medication	☐
Taking medications helps reduce certain distressing symptoms	☐	Continued symptoms despite medication	☐
Symptoms improved by medication	☐	Symptoms worsened by medication	☐
Medications help in maintaining stability	☐	Stopping medication does not lead to relapse or worsening of symptoms	☐
Medications prevent relapse	☐	Not in need of medication for relapse prevention	☐
Medications help with being more "normal"	☐	Medication interferes with being "normal"	☐
Side effects are better than those for other medications previously prescribed	☐	Side effect visible to others	☐
Medications help facilitate relationships with others	☐	Side effects interfere with functioning	☐
Medication has fewer side effects / patient does not feel "medicated"	☐	Distress over a side effect Fear of a future side effect	☐
Medication helps with achieving a life goal	☐	Medication interferes with achieving a life goal	☐
Patient is influenced by family/ friend to stay with medication	☐	Patient is influenced by family/friend to go off medication	☐
Patient is influenced by mental health clinician to stay with medication	☐	Relationship problems between mental health clinicians interfere with adherence	☐
Patient is not concerned about stigma of medication	☐	Patient feels stigmatized by medication	☐
If patient is using other drugs or alcohol, feels that staying on medication is useful during episodes of drug/substance use	☐	Patient is using other drugs or alcohol, stops medication during times of use	☐

Adapted from the Rating of Medication Influences assessment (Weiden, Rapkin, Mott, Zygmunt, Goldman, & Frances, 1994).

Relevance or importance can be rated as: score of 1 = present but minimal influence on adherence; 2 = some influence on adherence; and 3 = strong influence on adherence.

establishment of more adherence-congruent beliefs through examining the evidence for the belief and weighing advantages and disadvantages. It is also often useful to refer to an *adherence timeline over the course of the illness,* paying particular attention to relating adherence status to periods when the patient subjectively recalls feeling better on the one hand, and periods of increased symptomatology and distress, on the other hand.

Establish more adherence-congruent beliefs

Adherence timeline over the course of the illness

8.6.2. Education and Collaboration With Family and Carers

Table 24 suggests that family psychoeducation is a primary intervention for patients whose families are ambivalent or opposed to medication. It is important to keep in mind that a *CBT-oriented psychotherapy and family psychoeducation are perfectly compatible*; the kind of psychoeducation that may conflict with CBT is patient-based psychoeducation that relies on biomedical model explanations. Of course, family psychoeducation is more than an adherence intervention – outcomes are greatly improved when families are actively engaged in the treatment of schizophrenia. Families are also an *important source of information for clinicians about possible barriers to adherence* (Pitschel-Walz et al., 2006). As part of the adherence assessment process, it is very helpful to ask about who is influential within the person's support system, and to understand those individuals' beliefs and attitudes about medication. Families may have a wide range of opinions about antipsychotic medication.

CBT-oriented psychotherapy and family psychoeducation are perfectly compatible

Family-based psychoeducation is an evidence-based core intervention, and adherence is often a basic part of family work. Many of the principles reviewed in other aspects of this chapter can be applied to work with families (Rettenbacher, Burns, Kemmler, & Fleischhacker, 2004). Depending on the circumstances, *family work can be part of a CBT intervention,* using the same principles of problem lists and shared goals that are common to a CBT treatment plan.

8.6.3 Patient's Perspective on Medication Efficacy

Efficacy and adherence are closely linked. Just as poor adherence can lead to persistent symptoms, persistent symptoms can lead to poor adherence. For symptomatic patients, better symptom response generally translates to better long-term adherence (Hofer et al., 2007; Perkins et al., 2006, 2008). Persistent negative symptoms are a less consistent predictor. While negative symptoms can interfere with the patient's ability to take medication, sometimes the passivity associated with negative symptoms makes it difficult for the patient to act on their desire to stop medication. Should there be improvement in negative symptoms, then the patient may take action and stop medication. This example illustrates the clinical utility of assessing both adherence attitude as well as behavior. For the most part, however, there is a *correlation between better symptom control and better adherence,* and this extends to patient self-report of efficacy: Higher levels of perceived beneficial effects of medication are associated with reduced risk of early treatment discontinuation (Liu-Seifert, Adams, Ascher-Svanum, Faries, & Kinon, 2007; Liu-Seifert, Adams, & Kinon, 2005).

Correlation between better symptom control and better adherence

8.6.4   Distress From Side Effects

It is beyond the scope of this review to fully discuss all side effects. From a CBT perspective, it is the distress from perceived side effects that matters in terms of likelihood of creating adherence problems. In general, *prescribing clinicians may not be as aware of the impact of "minor" side effects* on the goals or priorities of the patient. This difference of opinion between patient and clinician perspectives, however, can be part of a normalizing process that might decrease the tension between the patient and the prescribing clinician. The *initial problem list can help identify key "hot" issues* where any perceived side effect can become a serious psychological impediment for the patient. For example, someone whose primary goal is to go back to work as a computer programmer may be very distressed by sedation, even if achieving that goal seems remote at the moment.

Also, for patients who are concerned about maintaining or developing a social network, *some side effects will be more disruptive than others.* A common example during acute treatment is when acute parkinsonism or akathisia is so upsetting to the family that they no longer support the doctor's recommendation for medication. Other common examples that may be more insidious and gradually erode support of others include persistent sedation, weight gain, sexual dysfunction, menstrual cycle disruption, and galactorrhea. Finally, if the patient perceives that the prescribing or the CBT clinician is not taking the distress seriously – regardless of whether the distress is warranted – it will probably be detrimental to the therapeutic engagement process. Alternatively, if *the patient feels that the clinician takes the concerns seriously,* this may strengthen the therapeutic engagement even when there is no immediate way to alleviate the perceived adverse effects.

A caveat is that the CBT approach discussed here is not comprehensive, and cannot substitute for a full medical assessment of safety issues related to antipsychotic medication. For example, medication-induced lipid abnormalities are rarely the cause of distress and yet are medically important. Likewise, tardive dyskinesia requires monitoring even though many patients will not be aware of any dyskinesia movements. Therefore, the approach to subjective distress from side effects used in a CBT-oriented adherence interview is meant to supplement, but not substitute for, ongoing medication safety assessments.

Prescribing clinicians may not be as aware of the impact of "minor" side effects

Some side effects will be more disruptive than others

9 Adapting CBT for Psychosis Strategies to Specific Patient Needs

Although CBT strategies were first evaluated for, and applied to, patients with chronic delusions and hallucinations only, there are no major objections to adapting these techniques to a variety of treatment settings as well as special needs with which patients may present in clinical practice. For example, CBT strategies can be helpful for first-episode psychosis patients coming into psychiatric treatment for the very first time and for dual-diagnosis patients requiring additional treatment components to address drug and/or alcohol use issues. The CBT clinician always chooses treatment strategies based on the individual patient's goals, and thus, these techniques can be adapted according to the patient's special needs. This flexibility of clinical practice in combination with a strong therapeutic relationship and the strong collaboration with and involvement of the patient, such as during the development and hierachization of a problem list as outlined in Section 4.1, constitute the primary foundations of CBT treatment of psychosis. In this chapter, however, we will discuss treatment aspects that may need special consideration for certain patient groups with specific needs.

9.1 First-Episode Psychosis

The initial onset of psychosis is usually preceded by a nonspecific prodromal period characterized by social withdrawal, social anxiety, depression, functional decline, and breakthrough intermittent psychotic symptoms prior to the manifestation of core schizophrenia symptoms such as hallucinations, delusions, disordered thinking, and emotional withdrawal. Recent efforts to better characterize illness prodrome and the transition to psychosis (Woods et al., 2009) along with findings that early treatment intervention may be associated with better functional outcome (McGorry, Killackey, & Yung, 2007) have brought a new importance to treatment strategies specific to patients in their first episode of psychotic illness.

Early intervention approaches include two elements that are distinctly different from standard care for chronic schizophrenia patients:

(1) early detection of people who are likely to develop psychosis and prevention of the onset of schizophrenia in people with prodromal symptoms and

Early intervention approaches

Table 26. Use of cognitive therapy in early intervention	
1. Valuable as an assessment tool for:	• Identifying "as if" issues • Delusional mood • Incipient passivity – "like being controlled" • "Perhaps" mechanisms
2. Role as therapeutic intervention with preventive role:	• Using normalization and instilling hope • Acceptability to the client's group • Possible to use in limiting transition to psychosis

> (2) effective phase-specific treatment for people in their first episode of psychosis with the goal of reducing the ultimate severity of the illness.

CBT for psychosis can be a valuable adjunct to early intervention strategies. Specifically, the collaborative and exploratory way of working with the patient can assist with the initial identification of psychotic symptoms and related stressors. CBT strategies that are especially useful in early intervention are summarized in Table 26 (Kingdon & Turkington, 2005).

Early intervention services are now widespread throughout America, Europe, and Australia (Marshall & Rathbone, 2006). Generally, the number of existing trials is still insufficient to draw definite conclusions about the effectiveness of specific early interventions for psychosis. One study showed that a combination of risperidone treatment and CBT can delay the manifestation of the first psychotic episode in people with prodromal symptoms by up to 6 months, although it remained unclear whether this effect was due to the risperidone treatment or the use of CBT strategies (McGorry et al., 2002). Another study showed no differences in transition rates to psychosis between patients treated with CBT and patients receiving supportive therapy (Morrison et al., 2002, 2004). Studies evaluating CBT for treatment of first-episode schizophrenia showed immediate large improvements in reduction of positive symptoms at short-term and mid-treatment follow-up in CBT treatment groups compared with those receiving treatment as usual, supportive therapy, or befriending (Drury, Birchwood, & Cochrane, 2000; Jackson et al., 2001, 2005, 2008; Morrison et al., 2004; Tarrier et al., 2004). However, these advantages of CBT have not been shown to be sustained at follow-up evaluations after 1 year or more (Drury et al., 2000; Jackson et al., 2001, 2005, 2008; Tarrier et al., 2004).

First episode of schizophrenia is a critically important time

For the patient, the *first episode of schizophrenia is a critically important time* that can decide the future course of illness and also constitutes a window of opportunity for timely, comprehensive, and effective therapeutic interventions. The hope is that proper management during this critical period can favorably influence the long-term trajectory of illness and functional outcome (Weiden, Buckley, & Grody, 2007). Shortening the duration of untreated psychosis is theoretically important in limiting the toxic effects of untreated psychotic symptoms on eventual treatment response. The use of CBT strategies as a valuable adjunct to early intervention programs can help achieve early recovery in patients experiencing their first episode of psychoses.

Table 27. Active CBT for early psychosis

• Assessment of presenting psychotic and nonpsychotic complaints
• Formulation of relationships between complaints and patient's life history
• Hierachization of problems:
  1. Any issue of risk
  2. Positive symptoms if present and distressing
  3. Comorbidities
  4. Negative symptoms
  5. Issues of identity
  6. Relapse prevention

Adapted from Jackson et al. (2008)

Incorporating CBT strategies into early intervention has several goals:
(1) encouragement of acceptability of the mental illness and motivation for treatment,
(2) reducing the loss of functioning due to illness as much as possible, and
(3) prevention of secondary psychiatric illness such as posttraumatic stress syndrome after compulsory hospitalization or treatment, substance abuse, social anxiety, or depression (Jackson et al., 2008).

To enhance the goal and expectation of optimal recovery, it is recommended that CBT is introduced to first-episode patients after medication treatment, clinical stabilization, and symptom remission have begun (Addington & Gleeson, 2005). An example of a CBT intervention for first-episode patients is given in Table 27.

The ongoing engagement of the first-episode patient in the therapeutic process is essential for the success of the intervention and must involve a flexible approach by the clinician to the timing, location, and content of therapy – e.g., it may include going for a bike ride.

Using CBT strategies in the treatment of first-episode psychosis patients requires the consideration of several issues that are distinctly different from aspects related to the treatment of chronically ill patients and that are unique to patients in the early course of illness.

In contrast to patients with a history of chronic illness, *first-episode patients are frequently not yet discouraged by previous treatment experiences,* so that establishing a therapeutic alliance characterized by acceptance and support may be easier for the clinician. However, first-episode patients are often overwhelmed by the exacerbation of acute psychotic symptoms and may not be used to clinical treatment routines. Consequently, they may show greater reservation toward the therapist than chronically ill patients. Additional reasons for negative attitudes toward treatment and clinicians may include internalized stigma about mental illness, a general avoidance of any health care providers, and most commonly, a lack of awareness about personal treatment needs. In this early phase, the *exploration of previous health care and therapeutic experiences* is vital for successful engagement and subsequent treatment success and thus becomes inevitable. Further, the identification of illness-related anxiety and depression is most important. As in the work with chronic patients, the use

Exploration of previous health care and therapeutic experiences

of normalizing is one important tool that can mediate understanding and acceptance of the patient's problems, especially in patients who present with anxiety and suspicion related to treatment.

Most first-episode patients being diagnosed with schizophrenia have gone through exhausting phases of transition during the prior months or even years. Patients have to make the significant adjustment from not having been formally treated in a mental health care system to being identified as a patient with a severe mental illness and receiving a recommendation for ongoing treatment. These *initial transitional phases are frightening and distressing for the patients and their families* and often leave them in a state of pure confusion. CBT strategies are effective in helping patients to develop a future perspective. Encouragement of joint problem-understanding by means of developing a personalized working model of the patient's symptoms and distress and the reduction of negative effects of the symptoms on self-image and self-esteem therefore represent primary goals for CBT strategies.

Depending on the length of the prodromal phase and the duration of untreated psychosis, *significant psychosocial damage* may already be part of first-episode patients' lives by the time they present to treatment for the very first time. Therefore, the goals for CBT strategies in first-episode schizophrenia patients must also include helping patients adapt to symptoms by improving role functioning at home, in school, or at work, and in social situations through the use of social skills training and help with age-appropriate resolutions of developmental tasks, such as emancipation from the parental household or the forming of romantic partnerships.

First-episode patients may be unwilling or unable to disclose the full extent of symptoms during the first therapy sessions, and family members may be too shocked or overwhelmed to fully report the severity or magnitude of existing problems. Therefore, therapists must keep in mind that the true nature of the course of illness will tend to unfold only over time (Weiden et al., 2007).

When initially evaluating a first-episode patient, it is important to *gain a functional understanding of present risk factors.* There has been a major shift from the previously accepted concept that the risk for developing schizophrenia arises primarily from a neurodevelopmental disorder. Recent research suggests that environmental factors, e.g., stressors, are the cause of the onset of the initial psychotic episode. The most important risk factors include urbanicity, social adversity, and marijuana exposure. The detailed assessment of these stressors, which presumably triggered the conversion of a genetic predisposition into a psychotic illness, as well as their impact on the individual, may be easier in first-episode patients than in chronically ill patients for whom the initial illness episode may have happened decades before.

Discussing the effects of stress within the context of the vulnerability–stress model, including personal aspects that induce individually perceived pressures for the patient, generally represents an acceptable approach for most patients when introducing psychoeducation. When stressors are identified in a joint effort with the patient, he or she is more likely to develop an intrinsically generated interest in reducing or coping with these stressors – e.g., by learning stress management techniques – which may also contribute to successful relapse prevention. In addition to personalized coping techniques, stress reduction strategies may also include advising patients to take time off from school or work

Initial transitional phases are frightening and distressing

Significant psychosocial damage

Gain a functional understanding of present risk factors

Discussing the effects of stress

and suggesting to caregivers that they "let go" – that is, to ease off and show their good intentions through support and simply being available, rather than asserting strong opinions and expectations (Kingdon & Turkington, 2005).

Following recovery from the first acute phase of psychosis, rates of patients who deny that they are ill are over 50% (Amador et al., 1994) and are thus higher than in chronically ill patients. Importantly, a *CBT approach does not require patient insight* but is rather based on the person's acceptance that he or she is stressed, unwell, and can benefit from treatment. There is evidence that increased acceptance of the need for treatment and recognition that voices or delusions are originating from within oneself both correlate positively with improved outcome (Kingdon & Turkington, 2005). It is not necessary to use the diagnostic term *schizophrenia* during psychoeducation work with patients. Rather, clinicians should attempt to use the descriptive terms defined by the patients when explaining their experiences in order to form a common and mutually understood and agreed upon language. Subsequently, CBT strategies seem to be ideal for building a therapeutic alliance with first-episode patients, who are not yet aware of their diagnosis or simply reject the diagnosis of schizophrenia.

Treatment of the very first episode of schizophrenia is of critical importance to patients, family members, and also clinicians because this initial experience will influence – for better or worse – the acceptance of ongoing treatment, including acceptance of medications, by the patient in the years ahead. Although acute symptoms usually respond well to antipsychotic treatment, less than 20% of a sample of first-episode psychosis patients were reported to take antipsychotic medication consistently throughout follow-up (Mojtabai, Lavelle, Gibson, & Bromet, 2003). Today, *nonadherence to medication* regimens is a greater obstacle to the successful treatment of first-episode schizophrenia than any other limitations in efficacy of the newer medications (Weiden et al., 2007). The nonadherence problem gains further importance particularly for first-episode patients because relapse in this group is associated with a higher suicide risk than in chronically ill patients. CBT strategies aim to overcome this problem by placing a greater emphasis on maintaining the therapeutic alliance at all times regardless of the patient's current adherence status. Such a long-term perspective may prevent initial nonadherence from becoming an established response to treatment options in the years to come. Recent studies show that nonpharmacologic factors such as the therapeutic alliance are much more relevant predictors for medication adherence than are side effects of medications (McEvoy et al., 2006). Accordingly, another study demonstrated that the majority of first-episode patients were accepting of long-acting antipsychotic medication when the treatment was mediated by a tailored intervention focusing on matching the goals of antipsychotic therapy to the long-term goals of the patient and family (Weiden, et al., 2006a).

In summary, when considering these issues that are somewhat specific to first-episode psychosis patients compared with chronically ill patients, it becomes apparent that CBT strategies represent valuable adjunct techniques to early intervention programs. They are especially important for establishing sustained therapeutic alliances and for introducing antipsychotic medication as one possible tool that can help patients reach their individual treatment goals.

9.2. Dual-Diagnosis Patients

Among chronically ill patients with schizophrenia living in the United States, 23% have reported nonproblematic substance use, but 37% have comorbid substance use disorders (Swartz et al., 2006). These patients are also often referred to as dual-diagnosis patients. Of patients with a substance use disorder, 87% report using alcohol, 44% use marijuana, and 36% use cocaine (Swartz et al., 2006). Although this study showed higher or equivalent overall social functioning scores in patients who used or abused cannabis or alcohol compared with abstinent patients, other studies have shown that even low levels of substance abuse or dependence represent a risk factor for serious complications, including suicide, poor compliance with treatment, more inpatients stays, violence, and poor overall prognosis (Barrowclough et al., 2001; Ridgely, Goldman, & Willenbring, 1990).

The management of dual-diagnosis issues in patients with schizophrenia begins with the assessment of both positive and negative consequences of the substance use. The decision whether *specific interventions for substance use* are needed depends on whether substance consumption is clearly associated with (a) repeated precipitation of psychotic episodes, (b) perpetuation of symptoms with continuing use of substances, (c) negative social consequences from drug consumption, or (d) whether the patient is unable to participate in any therapeutic work due to substance use effects (Kingdon & Turkington, 2005).

Treatment approaches for dual-diagnosis patients usually rely on *integrated programs*, most often combining motivational interviewing with individual CBT, and/or family or caregiver interventions (Barrowclough et al., 2001, 2009). An investigation of this approach in a randomized controlled trial showed significant improvements in patients' functioning compared with those receiving routine care, after 18 months of treatment (Haddock et al., 2003). Of note, no significant differences between treatment groups were found for caregiver and cost outcomes (Haddock et al., 2003). A recent systematic review of 54 studies investigating psychosocial treatments for co-occurring severe mental illness and substance misuse demonstrated that motivational interviewing showed the highest quality evidence for reducing substance abuse over short-term periods, and, when combined with CBT, improvements in mental state were also apparent; CBT alone, however, showed little consistent support (Cleary, Hunt, Matheson, & Walter, 2009).

The core features of CBT interventions within integrated programs for dual-diagnosis patients aim to establish a functional analysis of links between social, biological, and psychological vulnerabilities for psychosis and (a) consequences of the illness and (b) drug use. CBT strategies should be used to ameliorate chronic delusions and hallucinations (Barrowclough et al., 2001) and should facilitate patients in finding links between their substance use and problems achieving life goals, and consequently increase patients' awareness of necessary changes in their substance use pattern (Barrowclough et al., 2009). The goal is to promote alternate ways of coping and to encourage treatment adherence (Weiss et al., 2007).

The rationale for the *synthesis of motivational interviewing with CBT* and caregiver interventions is based on the assumptions that

Table 28. Integrated intervention program

First 5 weeks	Motivational interviewing designed to assess and enhance patient's motivation to change. Changes in substance use are negotiated on an individual basis by formulating a shared understanding of factors that need to be changed if the client is to achieve goals of personal importance. The building of this shared formulation is assisted by the understanding of the interactions between substance use and psychosis (Barrowclough et al., 2007). Instilling hope for a better future through learning alternative coping strategies may convince patients to agree to decrease their substance use, especially in those using substances for managing harmful psychotic symptoms.
From 6th week on (or earlier if appropriate)	Integration of motivational interviewing style into cognitive behavioral therapy (CBT) sessions both in the sense that motivational interviewing continues to permeate therapy, and also as a default style when motivational issues emerge (Miller & Rollnick, 2002). Where appropriate, a written change plan is collaboratively drawn up, summarizing agreed upon goals and strategies. Weekly CBT sessions should go through about 20 sessions and may include: • identifying and increasing awareness of high-risk situations/warning signs • developing new coping skills for handling such high-risk situations/warning signs, with particular attention to psychosis symptom– and mental health–related problems highlighted in the formulation (e.g., strategies for dealing with distressing voices or with depressed mood) • coping with cravings and urges • making lifestyle changes so as to decrease need/urges for drugs and/or alcohol or to increase healthy activities and alternative options to substance use; normalizing lapses in substance use and developing strategies and plans for acting in the event of lapse/relapse so that adverse consequences may be minimized • cognitive restructuring around alcohol and drug expectancies
For an additional 3 months	CBT sessions every other week
Caregiver sessions	Ten to 16 sessions should be provided to caregivers, e.g., family members, after a list of shared goals of patients and caregivers has been generated. These sessions can involve family members alone, or take the form of integrated family–patient sessions. Caregivers can be supportive, collusive, or can have mixed unhelpful, albeit understandable, attitudes and reactions. Thus, taking a negotiating approach with the caregivers when called on to provide support for the patient can be a successful strategy (Kingdon & Turkington, 2005)

Adapted from Barrowclough et al. (2001, 2009)

(1) most patients are unmotivated to change their substance use
(2) patients' schizophrenia symptoms might be a factor in the maintenance of substance use, but drug and alcohol use might exacerbate symptoms, and
(3) family stress might have a particularly detrimental effect on treatment outcomes of dual-diagnosis patients (Barrowclough et al., 2001).

An example of an integrated treatment intervention for dual-diagnosis patients with schizophrenia is summarized in Table 28. This 9- to 12-month program can take place in the caregiver's or patient's home.

When working with dual-diagnosis patients, some further aspects should be considered (Kingdon & Turkington, 2005):
(1) Patients who are using illicit drugs may be concerned about the therapist's attitude toward them and may feel anxious that it will be punitive. Thus, the assessment of the patient's experience with the illicit drug should be free of any judgment but rather focus on the fact that they may be particularly vulnerable to negative effects of (illicit) drugs.
(2) Such patients may be specifically prone to a worsening of paranoia or hallucinations triggered by the fear of getting arrested by the police or persecuted by a drug dealer.
(3) Patients with drug-induced first-episode psychotic symptoms may develop a protracted psychotic illness. It is important to provide ongoing support to these patients and their caregivers, although this can be frustrating in light of potential ongoing substance use. The essential message communicated by the clinician should be that interventions are readily available for these patients and their caregivers whenever they are ready to receive them. This can make efforts of continued engagement and long-term management much more successful.

9.3   CBT for Psychotic Symptoms Occurring in Disorders Other Than Schizophrenia

Although rare, chronic psychotic symptoms occurring in psychiatric conditions such as mood disorders, anxiety disorders, obsessive compulsive disorder, or personality disorders can persist despite antipsychotic treatment. When psychotic symptoms complicate the treatment of these primary disorders, *patients may benefit from CBT-based strategies for coping with positive symptoms*. CBT strategies may be used to enable patients to conceptualize symptoms such as "voices" as internal rather than external phenomena – i.e., voices being representations of their own thoughts – in order for psychotic symptoms to be better understood and subsequently recede (Kingdon & Turkington, 2005). Using this approach, CBT strategies for coping with chronic voices (see Chapter 5) can address the harmful content of voices, especially when they express a patient's negative self-image, which may be based on abusive, traumatic, or otherwise harmful previous experiences (Kingdon & Turkington, 2005). Addressing persistent psychotic symptoms by applying CBT strategies in such a manner can help the primary diagnosis to then become the major focus of the therapeutic work.

Patients may benefit from CBT-based strategies for coping with positive symptoms

9.4 Using CBT Strategies in Group Therapy Settings

Most often, CBT for psychosis is offered as an individual therapy intervention, allowing strategies and treatment steps to focus on the individual patient's goals. Using CBT strategies in group therapy may appear unreasonable since common goals established in a group setting may not sufficiently and effectively address individual patient needs. Also, sustained therapeutic alliance and emphasis on patient–clinician collaboration typical for the CBT approach may appear more easily achieved in an individual rather than a group setting. However, therapeutic processes such as *group coherence effects and the sharing of experiences are often highly beneficial* to, and valued by, patients and are obviously not part of the individual therapy experience. In fact, a few studies have demonstrated comparable effect sizes for group and individual CBT interventions (Wykes et al., 2008).

Group coherence effects and the sharing of experiences are often highly beneficial

For group therapy approaches in the treatment of persistent psychotic symptoms, enhanced supportive therapy consisting of CBT strategies in addition to supportive therapy elements appears to be a promising strategy. A recent randomized controlled trial compared the effectiveness of group CBT with that of enhanced group supportive therapy for the treatment of auditory hallucinations. Results showed that group CBT was associated with a reduction in psychotic symptoms throughout a 12-month follow-up, but not with a reduction in voice distress or intensity (Penn et al., 2009). Only participants who received enhanced supportive therapy, which aimed at increasing social integration, showed a reduction in negative beliefs about voices throughout the follow-up (Penn et al., 2009).

Group CBT strategies for reducing the negative impact of voices can include the following components (Penn et al., 2009; Wykes et al., 2005):

- Session 1:   Introduction and engagement
- Sessions 2 and 3: Psychoeducation
  Exploring models of psychosis
- Sessions 4 and 5: Sharing information about voices and their contents
  Discussing positive and negative experiences
- Sessions 6 and 7: Behavioral analysis of auditory hallucinations
  Exploring beliefs about voices
- Sessions 8 and 9: Exploring ameliorating and aggravating factors for auditory hallucinations, e.g., identifying situations that increase or decrease voices
- Sessions 10–12: Developing coping strategies for voices

Additional sessions may include strategies for improving self-esteem and can also be used as boosters for previously covered topics (Wykes et al., 2005).

In summary, available evidence on benefits of CBT group therapy for the treatment of psychosis is to date insufficient for meaningful conclusions about the effectiveness of this approach. *More research is needed* to differentiate CBT strategies useful in group therapy settings versus those treatment elements that are based on individual patient's goals and thus require the structure of individual therapy sessions.

More research is needed

9.5 Special Treatment Considerations: How to Deal With Treatment Obstacles

(1) Get supervision

Get supervision

As with every type of treatment, a range of difficulties or obstacles can occur when using a CBT approach for the treatment of patients with persistent psychotic symptoms. Principally, prior to using CBT strategies with this patient population, expert supervision should be guaranteed to assure effective and efficacious evidence-supported treatment, competent and timely feedback by experts throughout the course of treatment, as well as proper support in case of clinical crises.

(2) CBT differs from the traditional medical model

For most patients who have been treated for persistent psychotic symptoms, a CBT approach to their stressors and difficulties will represent a significant deviation from the treatment approaches with which they have become familiar. Specifically, the traditional medical model generally conceptualizes schizophrenia as a chronic brain disorder which will require most likely life-long medication intervention. Further, the relationship between the treating clinician and the patient is often characterized by a significant power differential, and the clinician is generally considered to be the knowledgeable expert who will make the treatment decisions he or she believes are best for the patient based on the clinician's training and experience. In contrast, a *CBT approach focuses on behavioral interventions* in addition to medication treatment and *emphasizes the collaborative relationship* between the patient and the clinician. The latter is reflected in

CBT approach focuses on behavioral interventions and emphasizes the collaborative relationship

(a) a collaborative treatment goal setting
(b) the negotiation of treatment particulars, including medications, based on the patient's previous experiences, concerns, and wishes
(c) the clinician's view of the patient as the primary expert on his or her symptom presentation and related distress and impairment in functioning.

While a CBT approach ultimately fosters the empowerment and active treatment involvement of patients, many patients may initially need repeated education about basics of the approach and encouragement to become appropriately involved.

(3) Alliance comes first

Alliance comes first

Generally speaking, with increasing positive or negative symptom severity, clinicians are required to pay especially close attention to maintaining the therapeutic alliance. While this is important in any therapy relationship, more acutely ill patients may experience greater difficulties trusting others, interpreting social interactions correctly, and counteracting emotional withdrawal and active social avoidance. Basic techniques such as engagement, befriending, and normalizing can prove very helpful in contributing to ongoing rapport and a therapeutic alliance with even the most impaired patients. When first engaging with a patient, clinicians should provide brief (10–15 min) sessions several times a week, which should be structured based on the patient's schedule, current difficulties and fears, personal interests, etc. Sometimes, establishing a therapeutic alliance can include leaving the office or ward environment, going for a walk with the patient, watching TV, etc. A frequent therapist error during the engagement phase is to try to move on too quickly before the patient is ready to engage in therapeutic work (Kingdon & Turkington, 2005).

(4) CBT requires active patient involvement

While patients generally enjoy and appreciate the active and engaged nature of CBT, many therapists face patients who have difficulties completing homework assignments. The practice of new skills and coping strategies, reality testing, as well as the completion of behavioral experiments is vital to the success of the therapy, and thus, patients will only be able to reap the full benefits of the treatment if they are able to participate fully. To minimize the possibility of homework avoidance, clinicians should make sure that all homework assignments:

- are mutually agreed upon and designed together with the patient
- are manageable and require only the type of resources that are easily available to the patient
- have been discussed within the context of a specific treatment goal to maximize patient understanding and patient investment in the assignment
- have been discussed in regards to potential positive and negative outcomes and the most likely associated cognitive and emotional responses of the patient
- are always reviewed and discussed in the next session as an integral part of the therapy

(5) Treatment goal discrepancies

Collaborative work in session on the treatment goal list is an essential part of the initial phase of CBT for psychotic disorders. When patient and therapist have different treatment goals, most often obstacles will occur. Therapists need to ensure that they have a very clear understanding of any delusional content that may underlie a patient's goals. What may appear to be a seemingly inconsequential goal in light of the severity of the psychosis may in fact be a superficial symptom of the underlying delusional system. For example, a therapist may not believe that being able to enjoy food is a worthwhile goal for an acutely psychotic patient and thus may ignore it. However, the underlying reason for the patient's inability to eat may be the paranoid delusion of all food being poisoned by intruders.

In general, whenever the therapeutic process appears to be halted by obstacles or active or passive patient resistance, clinicians should take the time to properly assess the underlying causes and dynamics. These may present as naturally occurring components of the therapeutic process, e.g., transference issues, but may also be matters that require more immediate actions, such as acute increases in psychotic symptoms or suicidal or homicidal ideations. If acute action such as an inpatient hospitalization is required, CBT treatment goals may temporarily need to be set aside until the safety of the patient and/ or others is assured, and the patient is again able to sufficiently engage in the treatment process. To maintain the therapeutic alliance, however, it may be beneficial to keep up with short contacts during the therapy break, e.g., the therapist may visit the patient while he or she is treated on an inpatient unit.

10   Case Examples

10.1   Case Example 1: Early Psychosis Work – The Importance of Engagement and Normalizing in Working with Difficult to Engage Early-Psychosis Patients

A 22-year-old woman presenting early in the course of schizophrenia was referred for a 16-week course of cognitive behavioral therapy (CBT) for psychosis treatment. The patient had seen her prescribing psychiatrist regularly since her first hospitalization approximately 2 years ago and had received one course of behavioral therapy. Her psychiatrist believed that she could benefit from CBT at this time due to increasing interpersonal difficulties between the patient and her family members and a general lack of future direction. The patient summarized her previous therapy experience as "useless" and expressed significant ambivalence about reengaging in talk therapy. However, she was willing to meet with the therapist to "see what he might have to offer."

During the first meeting with the therapist, the patient initially focused exclusively on her medication treatment, stating that she was unsatisfied with the limited level of effectiveness and the significant side effects. She was clearly used to restricting her discussions with clinicians to medication issues, and initially viewed the sessions with her CBT therapist as an extension of her medication management meetings. Interestingly, she had developed rather illustrative and precise ways of communicating the specifics of her frustrations, such as "I feel like I have a blanket over my brain. The meds make me stand still, but I want to move. I know that something is wrong, but I am not being treated for it." These statements showed the therapist that the patient possessed the ability to be perceptive and introspective – both very useful skills for fully benefiting from CBT. The patient also shared her sadness and helplessness over what she perceived to be preconceived notions about her held by her prescriber. Specifically, the patient had a history of substance abuse, and due to her frequent requests for changes in medication because of persistent symptoms, she was characterized as medication seeking. She was able to share with the therapist that she not only felt frustrated by this but more importantly did not feel listened to or taken seriously by her prescriber, resulting in profound feelings of lack of control over her treatment management.

In general, the patient appeared as very hopeless, disinterested, and disengaged from her treatment and recovery process, as illustrated in her statement "I've thrown in the towel. I just don't care anymore." Her early experiences with the mental health care system had formed and reinforced the impression that her illness had to be managed by professional experts only and that she was unable to make significantly important contributions to discussions regarding her treatment planning other than reporting on medication side effects. Because of the emphasis on medication treatment by her psychiatrist, she was also skeptical regarding the usefulness and effectiveness of other treatment modalities, such as CBT.

Focusing primarily on the goal to engage the patient, the therapist centered his initial responses on empathetic and normalizing statements, without pushing the patient to evaluate the accuracy or the extremes of her comments. His replies conveyed to the patient that he genuinely believed her distress and frustration, and also communicated the strong desire to fully understand her circumstances and struggles.

When asked about her current living situation and existing support network, the patient also shared difficulties in her interpersonal relationships with her primary social contacts. According to the patient, her mother would like her to move out of the house as soon as possible and had stated this to the patient numerous times, including in front of her prescriber, which made the patient feel ganged up on and isolated. Further, the patient's mother considered her difficult and lazy and generally appeared to have a hard time empathizing with the patient's situation, symptoms, and related challenges and frustrations. Due to the patient's previous drug abuse problem, her mother no longer trusted her and often conceptualized her difficulties in the context of drug use, accusing the patient of relapse. As one result, the mother had been managing the patient's limited income (she received a small monthly disability check) against the patient's will. However, because the patient lived in the mother's home and thus was expected to pay a certain amount for rent and food, she eventually had agreed to the arrangement. This was also a great source of frustration for the patient and constituted another area in her life she was not only unable to control but also fostered a sense of dependency and inability to make her own decisions. Her subsequent self-defeating attitude was reflected in comments like "I always do something wrong" and "Nobody ever tells me anything about what's going on with me."

These comments were very helpful for the therapist as they provided wonderful avenues for engaging the patient. During a brief explanation of what the patient could expect from therapy, he emphasized the importance for many people, not just patients, of having a safe, confidential environment in which one can talk about any challenges and frustrations without the worry of being judged or reprimanded. In other words, it is impossible to fail as a therapy patient. He further explained that he would not share the content of their conversations with anyone else, including her parents or other mental health care providers. As a second important point, the therapist started to work on instilling some hope in the patient. Not using her as an example, but continuing to speak generally, he explained that therapy is a somewhat unusual, but also unique and often enjoyable experience. While it is certainly unusual to open up to a complete stranger, it is also wonderful to speak with someone who does not have any previous knowledge about oneself and thus no previous impressions or preconceived notions, but who fills the role of a listener, confidant, and advocate. These comments aimed to introduce the idea to the patient that the therapist would not automatically take on her mother's or prescriber's opinions, but would consider her the primary source of information about her person, her behavior, and her circumstances.

Responding to the patient's feelings of hopelessness and isolation, the therapist casually asked whether or not she was familiar with anyone else who was living with schizophrenia. In this context, he mentioned that quite a few celebrities were also people who were living with mental illnesses, and shared a list of these famous individuals and their achievements. As is typical, the patient was very interested in this list and also quite surprised about some of the folks included. Not only did this illustrate to the patient that people are able to excel and succeed in life despite having a mental illness, but it also showed her that one does not have to be identified by the illness.

At the end of the session, the patient agreed to see her therapist again and negotiated an initial agreement of three more sessions. During this negotiation, her therapist stated that neither he nor the patient can know whether or not therapy would be helpful to the patient at all; however, the only way to find out would be to try. He also explained that not everyone was willing to try, which was perfectly acceptable, but his experience had been that most people ended up liking the process. He reiterated that it was completely up to the patient to decide whether or not she would like to come back. Regardless of her decision, he thanked her for coming in and giving him the chance to get to know her. If she decided not to return, there would be no hard feelings and certainly no negative consequences. She was going to make the decision whether or not to make therapy part of her treatment – independent of anyone else's wishes.

Additionally, the therapist explained that the schedule of sessions could be built around the patient's availability. Because often new therapy patients will feel overwhelmed by weekly sessions, it is beneficial to initially offer a flexible session model and share the control over the frequency and length of the sessions with the patient. In this case, the therapist offered the patient to make the decision about what day she would like to come in, how frequently she would like her visits to be (weekly versus every other week), and for how long she would like to meet (20 min initially versus 30 min versus 45 min). At the same time, the therapist stated that there are certainly circumstances that could happen to anyone under which appointments might have to be canceled or rescheduled, and regardless of how frequently this may have to happen, there would be no repercussions for not showing up to sessions, and therapy would not be terminated based on a no-show record. By reassuring the patient in this manner, the therapist gave the control over the session schedule fully over to the patient. This was a new experience for her, which helped build rapport and her interest in continuing her treatment relationship with the therapist. Additionally, it conveyed to her that sometimes seemingly established processes can change unexpectedly when trying new approaches to a challenge, e.g., trying a new type of therapy.

The therapist's flexibility about schedule, session content, etc., was a must with this patient early in the course of illness. She was not a "seasoned patient" and thus lacked the experience of what was expected of her, but also how useful different components of mental health care could be to her. Thus, it was the therapist's responsibility to carefully engage the patient and provide above all a *positive* treatment experience for her, to increase the chances that she would continuously seek proper help over the course of her illness when needed.

The patient attended sessions as agreed to with the therapist with a limited no-show record and number of cancellations. Through ongoing engagement and carefully guided exploration, she was able to collaborate with her therapist in setting treatment goals in the fourth session, which reflected her desire to be taken seriously as a person whose opinions, wishes, and arguments were well considered and respected. Using CBT techniques such as normalizing, Socratic questioning, and inference chaining while building on the patient's existing strengths, the therapist was able to permanently provoke meaningful change in the patient's self-defeating convictions over the course of therapy. Rather than thinking of herself as an invalid and unimportant communication partner, and as not having control over her life decisions and choices, the patient became more and more empowered, and her self-confidence increased to the degree that she was able to express her wishes effectively when communicating with others, including her mother and her prescribing psychiatrist.

10.2 Case Example 2: Chronic Patient Work – Giving the "Hopeless" Long-Term Patient New Perspectives

A 45-year-old man was referred by his prescribing psychiatrist for a course of cognitive behavioral therapy (CBT) in the hope that talk therapy might help the patient interact with others. Other than his prescriber, whom the patient saw every 2 to 3 months for regular medication management appointments, the patient had no social contacts to speak of due to severe paranoia and persecutory delusions that remained medication treatment resistant. Although these delusional convictions consumed much of the patient's thinking, he significantly suffered from his social isolation and thus agreed to "try out" talk therapy as a possible avenue to practice speaking with someone other than his prescriber. The patient initially negotiated with his psychiatrist that he would not have to commit to any length of treatment but could stop at any time, even after the first session, should he not like the therapist or therapy. Of note, over his nearly 30-year history of living with schizophrenia, a number of courses of different talk therapies had been started with the patient that all ended prematurely due to the patient dropping out or the therapists ending treatment early because of the high level of aggression with which the patient presented. In fact, the referring clinician offered the CBT therapist, who was female, the option of refusing the referral because in the past, all other female therapists had declined to work with the patient due to his intrusive and forceful behaviors and attitudes.

Knowing the patient's distrust of others, his previous negative treatment experiences, and the related potential difficulties of engagement, the therapist requested from the prescribing psychiatrist to ask the patient for permission for the therapist to call the patient at a specific day and time to introduce herself. During this brief phone conversation, the therapist negotiated with the patient to come in for a one-time meet-and-greet visit (not an official session), during which they could meet face-to-face and decide whether or not working together could benefit the patient in any way. By approaching the patient in this relaxed, nonthreatening, and nondirective way, he not only was given control over treatment choices, but was reassured that his wishes and opinions mattered and at the same time was introduced to the concept of collaborative decision-making.

The initial meet-and-greet visit focused entirely on engaging the patient. Specifically, the therapist exclusively asked process questions with the goal to make the patient feel comfortable and also to convey the sense that the therapist was well aware of the potential discomfort the patient must feel when meeting a new clinician. Using the normalizing technique, the therapist asked process questions like: "I can imagine that it might feel uncomfortable sitting down with a complete stranger to speak about your life and your thoughts. Do you feel like that right now?" and "If I were in your situation, I'd probably be worried that the therapist might want to know things about me that I am not willing to talk about and then perhaps get mad at me for refusing to answer all questions. Has this ever happened to you, and are you worried that I might do this?" This approach provided the patient with a sense of security by validating any resistant feelings he might have, and also gave him indirect permission to deny certain information until he was ready to share with the therapist, if that was ever the case. The patient responded very positively to the therapist, and when asked whether or not he experienced any difficulties or challenges in life that he might want to talk about in a therapy context, he expressed the wish to return for future sessions. The therapist suggested starting with shorter meetings than the usual 45-minute sessions, to give the patient ample time to get used to being in therapy, to which he agreed. This also served the purpose of avoiding the patient feeling overwhelmed or developing paranoia about the therapist over more information being shared in early sessions due to more time spent together.

The first few sessions were spent discussing the patient's current difficulties and frustrations. He explained his belief that all others always discriminate against him due to his minority status (patient was an African immigrant) and due to having a mental illness. He denied experiencing any positive interaction in many years, including with his prescribing doctor who he believed was "corrupt like all doctors". However, he depended on him for his prescriptions, which he felt helped with insomnia and anxiety, and thus continued to see him. The patient's preferred compensatory behavior was avoidance of social situations, which directly led to his current social isolation. He had become hypervigilant about the few interactions he had, e.g., going to the post office, and in an effort to proactively protect himself from discriminatory acts, he often approached interactions in an aggressive manner, in turn provoking others to respond accordingly. The patient considered these defensive and often negative responses as evidence that people truly are racist and discriminating against him, reinforcing his delusional conviction.

Most infuriating for the patient was his belief that his siblings were also very disrespectful toward him. He believed that they were acting against him in collaboration with his doctor, citing past involuntary hospitalizations initiated by family members and his prescriber as evidence of their ill will toward him. As a result, he had had no contact with most of his family members in the past 2 years with the exception of one sister who infrequently stopped by his apartment to drop off groceries and check on him.

In an effort to carefully build familiarity with the CBT approach of introducing some doubt into delusional convictions, the therapist used Socratic questioning to ask about some seemingly inconsistent parts of the patient's story, while continuously normalizing the patient's experiences and fears and paying close attention to using the patient's language when paraphrasing his thoughts:

> I can't even imagine how frustrating and scary it must be for you to feel that you cannot trust anybody and constantly have to be on guard to protect yourself from others. I would feel very upset and also often exhausted. I have one quick question, though, because I want to make sure that I really understand what you are going through. You said earlier that even your sisters and your doctor are racists and hate you. What confuses me is that I thought your siblings have the same race that you have, and as you know, your doctor also belongs to a racial minority. Perhaps I misunderstood you earlier, but could you bear with me and explain one more time how they are racists when it comes to you, even though they are all members of minority groups?

This conveyed to the patient that the therapist had empathy for his situation and genuine concern, but also introduced him to the idea that while the therapist will believe his convictions, the patient will have to logically explain his reasoning, and thus potentially adjust his beliefs should his initial logic not hold.

Through conversations like this one, the patient slowly started to not only become used to the therapist asking questions that were challenging him to take a new look at his beliefs, but also to move away from his black-and-white thinking and consider multiple explanations for people's behaviors. As much as possible, this was done in a very relaxed and enjoyable atmosphere. Also, in the beginning of therapy, the therapist purposely was "paranoid with the patient" and took his experiences at face value, while taking care not to reassure the patient's delusional convictions, but rather comment in very general ways and continue to normalize. This helped built trust and gain the most complete picture of the patient's day-to-day perceptual and especially emotional experiences without premature case conceptualization or attempts at cognitive remediation.

As part of the first few sessions, the patient was also encouraged to decide on a goal list for therapy. Reflecting his distress over his social isolation despite his paranoid and persecutory convictions, he stated, "I want to be able to better relate to people. And I want to talk more to people." The therapist validated his wishes and explored together with the patient possible avenues for how he might begin to reach these goals, continuously encouraging the patient and reminding him how well he was able to speak to the therapist in session. The patient mentioned a neighbor who he admired for being a great athlete, and he decided to say hello and ask about the neighbor's bicycle the next time he saw him as a first attempt at a social interaction. The therapist and patient worked together to think through different possible responses from the neighbor, including positive replies (neighbor returns the greeting and answers the patient's question in a friendly manner) and negative replies (neighbor ignores patient or responds rudely). By choosing this relatively simple task that most likely would not result in a negative experience for the patient (and it did not), the patient was able to build confidence in interacting with others and also started making experiences that represented counterevidence for his delusional convictions, which was discussed during the following session.

Later sessions focused on continued work on the patient's beliefs and generating alternative hypotheses for negative behaviors of others that he believed were directed at him. What was important for the patient during these discussions was the recognition on the therapist's end that some of his experiences were in fact negative and as such perceived correctly by the patient. Such examples were used to generate various hypotheses about the intentions and thought processes of people (other than the patient's paranoid ideations of racism and discrimination), and to discuss possible acceptable response behaviors other than aggression, as used by the patient in the past. Further, these cases were used as learning experiences to impress upon the patient that his expectations may not always be met by others, potentially resulting in disappointment or frustration on his end, but being independent of him as a person. Throughout this process, the patient's responses were continuously validated, normalized, and if necessary, questioned and evaluated. The last two were always done in collaboration with the patient using Socratic questioning and inference chaining.

Over the course of treatment, the patient became more and more open in therapy and shared more of his feelings and worries, specifically related to his personal lack of self-esteem and internalized stigma about his minority status and mental illness. Initially frequent statements such as "All white people are stupid" or "All white people are racist" became more infrequent and moved away from general statements to more specific complaints in reference to particular experiences – e.g., "When I went to the community college last week to register for classes, two girls looked at me, pointed at my shoes and laughed." Additionally, the patient was encouraged to think of characteristics he had in common with others in order to build a sense of connection and common experience, rather than only focusing the cognitive restructuring on adaptive explanations for negative behavior of others.

During the second half of the CBT course, the patient initiated more frequent contact with some of his siblings, starting with more frequent phone calls focused on enjoyable topics and eventually including visits for family occasions such as birthdays and holidays. He expressed great pleasure over these changes and felt more accepted by his siblings than before. He also successfully continued to work on his cognitive flexibility by challenging his black-and-white thinking and questioning automatic thoughts related to his previously very fixed delusional beliefs. While these beliefs did not completely disappear, he was certainly no longer severely distressed and socially isolated.

Treatment was terminated after 20 sessions. At this time, the patient had enrolled in college courses at a community college with the goal of finishing his degree in physics. Also, he went on a 2-week out-of-state trip with two of his sisters to visit a sick family member. After his return, he reported having had a wonderful time, feeling well-accepted, and being hopeful about a future positive and close relationship with his family. The patient described his therapy experience as very positive. At no time during treatment did he act out in an aggressive way beyond the typical and appropriate frustrations when discussing challenging topics. Two years after treatment termination, the patient's prescribing physician provided the therapist with an update: The patient had not been rehospitalized since his course of CBT and continued to do well. He was still attending college courses and was in regular contact with his family. In fact, family members still asked about specifics regarding the treatment that had given them back their brother.

10.3   Case Example 3: Adherence Work – Using the Health Belief Dialogue to Understand Patients' Medication Adherence Behaviors and Attitudes

A 28-year-old man started a 12-session program of cognitive behavioral therapy (CBT) for psychosis. He had had a characteristic relapse that seemed related to stress from returning to school, or possible nonadherence with a complicated regimen of several antipsychotic medications. In his history, his medication adherence was, at best, haphazard, and it seemed likely that nonadherence was a contributing factor to recurrent relapses and rehospitalizations. The patient did not consider relapse or rehospitalization to be a problem.

Medications and adherence were not discussed during the initial goal-setting sessions. His initial treatment goals were

(1) to have the therapy help him be more "upbeat" about life, and

(2) to be better able to "look forward to things that make me happy."

At first, none of these initial goals appeared to be related to medication; however, it seemed likely that his attitudes about medications would come up later on as treatment continued. During the third session, he was eager to discuss his life and its many hardships. His medication regimen was still unmentioned by him, but his therapist asked whether his medications had anything to do with any of his problems or dissatisfaction with life. This question was quickly brushed off and not pursued by either party. By Session 4, additional information relating to his initial goals emerged. The problems that formed the basis of his goals for CBT were discovered to be a result of feelings of self-hatred because he considered himself to be a "failure," which kept him from feeling "upbeat." Further, he struggled with constant misery from anxiety caused by his belief that his landlord was persecuting him. These problems were identified as being similar to longstanding difficulties that kept him from completing his high school education and were added to a revised list of treatment goals.

At the fifth session, a health belief dialogue assessment using the Adherence Attitude Interview was done, and the information gathered guided the discussion to how medications may have helped or interfered with his life. His attitudes and beliefs about the role of antipsychotic medications in his life were now reviewed in some detail. The clinician asked all questions about medications in a curious, nonjudgmental manner, specifically paying attention to understanding the patient's personal beliefs or circumstances that might facilitate or hinder medication adherence. The responses to the health belief dialogue revealed that the patient would deliberately withhold important information in his medical evaluations concerning his symptoms. His adherence would fluctuate widely because he could not tolerate the inconsistencies and ambiguities of his doctors' recommendations. Consequently, he would try to make medication decisions on his own.

Between Sessions 5 and 8, the patient was able to report how he had been devastated by the limitations of psychiatric medications. When he first came to a psychiatrist as a symptomatic teenager, he had felt that the benefits of medications had been "overpromised" by his prescribing doctors. He had hoped medication would completely resolve all symptoms and felt that his doctors went along with this unrealistic hope so that "he wouldn't get upset and just continue with the medication." Later, he felt misled by his doctors' "excessive enthusiasm" about medication benefits. As a response, the patient decided that it was better to manage his medications by himself since doctors were not reliable or trustworthy. He decided to follow some of the medication recommendations some of the time, as a kind of compromise to deal with the conflicting advice given by various clinicians.

This narrative information was obtained over three sessions, and once clarified, made it much easier to understand the patient's haphazard adherence in his recent past, illustrating the importance of not only tracking adherence behavior but especially adherence attitude from the patient's perspective, which do not necessarily have to match. The next session focused on a discussion about how people learn to move on in life despite disappointments. Finally, the clinician led the patient in a guided discussion on how to apply this lesson to obtaining potential benefits from medications even when they were limited in their effectiveness, without using threatening and fear-provoking statements like "If you don't take medications, you are sure to relapse." On his own, the patient came to understand the possible benefits that ongoing medication adherence might offer in helping him cope with his feelings of self-hatred and anxiety from his ongoing delusional fears. As his attitudes about medication changed, the patient finished his General Educational Development (GED) requirements for high school. He became much more consistent in taking his medications than he had been in the past. At 1-year follow-up, his family reported that his improvements were sustained and that he was still doing better than he had in many years.

References

Addington, J., & Gleeson, J. (2005). Implementing cognitive-behavioural therapy for first-episode psychosis. *The British Journal of Psychiatry Supplement, 48*, s72–76.

Aguglia, E., Pascolo-Fabrici, E., Bertossi, F., & Bassi, M. (2007). Psychoeducational intervention and prevention of relapse among schizophrenic disorders in the Italian community psychiatric network. *Clinical Practice and Epidemiology in Mental Health, 3*(7), 1–12.

Ajzen, I. (2001). Nature and operation of attitudes. *Annual Review of Psychology, 52*, 27–58.

Alam, D. A., & Janicak, P. G. (2005). The role of psychopharmacotherapy in improving the long-term outcome of schizophrenia. *Essential Psychopharmacology, 6*(3), 127–140.

Amador, X. F., Flaum, M., Andreasen, N. C., Strauss, D. H., Yale, S. A., Clark, S. C., et al. (1994). Awareness of illness in schizophrenia and schizoaffective and mood disorders. *Archives of General Psychiatry, 51*(10), 826–836.

American Psychiatric Association Steering Committee. (2004). *Practice guidelines for the treatment of patients with schizophrenia.* Arlington, VA: American Psychiatric Press.

Anderson, C. M., Hogarty, G. E., & Reiss, D. J. (1980). Family treatment of adult schizophrenic patients: A psycho-educational approach. *Schizophrenia Bulletin, 6*(3), 490–505.

Ba, M. B., Zanello, A., Varnier, M., Koellner, V., & Merlo, M. C. (2008). Deficits in neurocognition, theory of mind, and social functioning in patients with schizophrenic disorders: Are they related? *The Journal of Nervous and Mental Disease, 196*(2), 153–156.

Barrowclough, C., Haddock, G., Beardmore, R., Conrod, P., Craig, T., Davies, L., et al. (2009). Evaluating integrated MI and CBT for people with psychosis and substance misuse: Recruitment, retention and sample characteristics of the MIDAS trial. *Addictive Behaviors, 34*(10), 859–866.

Barrowclough, C., Haddock, G., Tarrier, N., Lewis, S. W., Moring, J., O'Brien, R., et al. (2001). Randomized controlled trial of motivational interviewing, cognitive behavior therapy, and family intervention for patients with comorbid schizophrenia and substance use disorders. *The American Journal of Psychiatry, 158*(10), 1706–1713.

Barrowclough, C., Haddock, G., Tarrier, N., Lewis, S. W., Moring, J., O'Brien, R., et al. (2007). Psychosis & Drug and Alcohol Problems. In Baker & Vellerman (Eds.), *Clinical handbook of co-existing mental health and drug and alcohol problems* (pp. 241–265). New York, and East Sussex, UK: Routledge.

Bäuml, J., & Pitschel-Walz, G. (2003). *Psychoedukation bei schizophrenen Erkrankungen: Konsensuspapier der Arbeitsgruppe „Psychoedukation bei schizophrenen Erkrankungen".* Stuttgart, Germany: Schattauer.

Bäuml, J., Pitschel-Walz, G., Volz, A., Engel, R. R., & Kessling, W. (2007). Psychoeducation in schizophrenia: 7-year follow-up concerning rehospitalization and days in hospital in the Munich Psychosis Information Project Study. *The Journal of Clinical Psychiatry, 68*(6), 854–861.

Bell, M., Bryson, G., Greig, T., Corcoran, C., & Wexler, B. E. (2001). Neurocognitive enhancement therapy with work therapy: Effects on neuropsychological test performance. *Archives of General Psychiatry, 58*(8), 763–768.

Bell, M., Tsang, H. W., Greig, T. C., & Bryson, G. J. (2009). Neurocognition, social cognition, perceived social discomfort, and vocational outcomes in schizophrenia. *Schizophrenia Bulletin, 35*(4), 738–747.

Ben-Yishay, Y., & Diller, L. (1993). Cognitive remediation in traumatic brain injury: Update and issues. *Archives of Physical Medicine and Rehabilitation, 74*(2), 204–213.

Bilder, R. M., Bogerts, B., Ashtari, M., Wu, H., Alvir, J. M., Jody, D., et al. (1995). Anterior hippocampal volume reductions predict frontal lobe dysfunction in first episode schizophrenia. *Schizophrenia Research, 17*(1), 47–58.

Brabban, A., Tai, S., & Turkington, D. (2009). Predictors of outcome in brief cognitive behavior therapy for schizophrenia. *Schizophrenia Bulletin, 35*(5), 859–864.

Brent, B. K., & Giuliano, A. J. (2007). Psychotic-spectrum illness and family-based treatments: A case-based illustration of the underuse of family interventions. *Harvard Review of Psychiatry, 15*(4), 161–168.

Burton, S. (2006). Symptom domains of schizophrenia: The role of atypical antipsychotic agents. *Journal of Psychopharmacology (Oxford, England), 20*(6 Suppl), 6–19.

Butzlaff, R. L., & Hooley, J. M. (1998). Expressed emotion and psychiatric relapse: a meta-analysis. *Archives of General Psychiatry, 55*(6), 547–552.

Carpenter, W. T., & Conley, R. R. (2007). Challenge to atypical antipsychotic drug effect on cognition. *The American Journal of Psychiatry, 164*(12), 1910–1911; author reply 1911–1912.

Carroll, A., Fattah, S., Clyde, Z., Coffey, I., Owens, D. G., & Johnstone, E. C. (1999). Correlates of insight and insight change in schizophrenia. *Schizophrenia Research, 35*(3), 247–253.

Carter, D. M., Mackinnon, A., & Copolov, D. L. (1996). Patients' strategies for coping with auditory hallucinations. *The Journal of Nervous and Mental Disease, 184*(3), 159–164.

Cleary, M., Hunt, G. E., Matheson, S., & Walter, G. (2009). Psychosocial treatments for people with co-occurring severe mental illness and substance misuse: Systematic review. *Journal of Advanced Nursing, 65*(2), 238–258.

Coleman, R., & Smith, M. (1997). Accepting and beginning to live with voices. In *Working with voices: Victim to victor* (pp. 37–43). Stockport, UK: Handsell Publishing

Coleman, R., & Smith, M. (2003). *Working with voices: Victim to victor.* (2nd ed.) Fife, UK: P&P Press.

Conner, M., Povey, R., Sparks, P., James, R., & Shepherd, R. (2003). Moderating role of attitudinal ambivalence within the theory of planned behaviour. *The British Journal of Social Psychology 42*(Pt 1), 75–94.

Cunningham Owens, D. G., Carroll, A., Fattah, S., Clyde, Z., Coffey, I., & Johnstone, E. C. (2001). A randomized, controlled trial of a brief interventional package for schizophrenic out-patients. *Acta Psychiatrica Scandinavica, 103*(5), 362–369.

David, A. S. (1990). Insight and psychosis. *The British Journal of Psychiatry, 156*, 798–808.

Davidson, M., Galderisi, S., Weiser, M., Werbeloff, N., Fleischhacker, W. W., Keefe, R. S., et al. (2009). Cognitive effects of antipsychotic drugs in first-episode schizophrenia and schizophreniform disorder: A randomized, open-label clinical trial (EUFEST). *The American Journal of Psychiatry, 166*(6), 675–682.

DiClemente, C. C., Bellino, L. E., & Neavins, T. M. (1999). Motivation for change and alcoholism treatment. *Alcohol Research & Health, 23*(2), 86–92.

Draper, M. L., Stutes, D. S., Maples, N. J., & Velligan, D. I. (2009). Cognitive adaptation training for outpatients with schizophrenia. *Journal of Clinical Psychology, 65*(8), 842–853.

Drury, V., Birchwood, M., & Cochrane, R. (2000). Cognitive therapy and recovery from acute psychosis: A controlled trial: Part 3: Five-year follow-up.*The British Journal of Psychiatry, 177*, 8–14.

Drury, V., Birchwood, M., Cochrane, R., & Macmillan, F. (1996). Cognitive therapy and recovery from acute psychosis: A controlled trial: Part I: Impact on psychotic symptoms. *The British Journal of Psychiatry, 169*(5), 593–601.

Eack, S. M., Hogarty, G. E., Greenwald, D. P., Hogarty, S. S., & Keshavan, M. S. (2007). Cognitive enhancement therapy improves emotional intelligence in early course schizophrenia: Preliminary effects. *Schizophrenia Research, 89*(1–3), 308–311.

Ehlers, A. (1999). *Posttraumatische Belastungsstoerungen.* Goettingen, Germany: Hogrefe.

Eickhoff, K., Vauth, R., & Olbrich, H. M. (1997). Streß-/Angst-Management und Selbstkonzeptstabilisierung bei persistierender Wahnsymptomatik. In C. Mundt, M. Linden & W. Barnett (Eds.), *Psychotherapie in der Psychiatrie* (pp. 101–108). Berlin, Germany: Springer Verlag.

Falkai, P., Wobrock, T., Lieberman, J., Glenthoj, B., Gattaz, W. F., & Moller, H. J. (2006). World Federation of Societies of Biological Psychiatry (WFSBP) guidelines for biological treatment of schizophrenia: Part 2: Long-term treatment of schizophrenia. *World Journal of Biological Psychiatry, 7*(1), 5–40.

Falloon, I. R. H., Boyd, J. L., & McGill, C. W. (1984). *Family care for schizophrenia: A problem-solving treatment for mental illness.* New York, NY: Guilford Press.

Fenton, W. S. (2000). Evolving perspectives on individual psychotherapy for schizophrenia. *Schizophrenia Bulletin, 26*(1), 47–72.

Frank, A. F., & Gunderson, J. G. (1990). The role of the therapeutic alliance in the treatment of schizophrenia: Relationship to course and outcome. *Archives of General Psychiatry, 47*(3), 228–236.

Garety, P., Fowler, D., Kuipers, E., Freeman, D., Dunn, G., Bebbington, P., et al. (1997). London-East Anglia randomised controlled trial of cognitive-behavioural therapy for psychosis: Part II: Predictors of outcome. *The British Journal of Psychiatry, 171*, 420–426.

Ginsberg, D. L., Schooler, N. R., Buckley, P. F., Harvey, P. D., & Weiden, P. J. (2005). Optimizing treatment of schizophrenia: Enhancing affective/cognitive and depressive functioning. *CNS Spectrums, 10*(2), 1–13; discussion 14–15.

Gold, J. M., & Harvey, P. D. (1993). Cognitive deficits in schizophrenia. *The Psychiatric Clinics of North America, 16*(2), 295–312.

Goldberg, T. E., Hyde, T. M., Kleinman, J. E., & Weinberger, D. R. (1993). Course of schizophrenia: Neuropsychological evidence for a static encephalopathy. *Schizophrenia Bulletin, 19*(4), 797–804.

Green, M. F. (1996). What are the functional consequences of neurocognitive deficits in schizophrenia? *The American Journal of Psychiatry, 153*(3), 321–330.

Green, M. F., Kern, R. S., Braff, D. L., & Mintz, J. (2000). Neurocognitive deficits and functional outcome in schizophrenia: Are we measuring the "right stuff"? *Schizophrenia Bulletin, 26*(1), 119–136.

Green, M. F., & Nuechterlein, K. H. (1999). Should schizophrenia be treated as a neurocognitive disorder? *Schizophrenia Bulletin, 25*(2), 309–319.

Gumley, A., O'Grady, M., McNay, L., Reilly, J., Power, K., & Norrie, J. (2003). Early intervention for relapse in schizophrenia: Results of a 12-month randomized controlled trial of cognitive behavioural therapy. *Psychological Medicine, 33*(3), 419–431.

Haddock, G., Barrowclough, C., Tarrier, N., Moring, J., O'Brien, R., Schofield, N., et al. (2003). Cognitive-behavioural therapy and motivational intervention for schizophrenia and substance misuse: 18-month outcomes of a randomised controlled trial. *The British Journal of Psychiatry, 183*, 418–426.

Haddock, G., Slade, P. D., Bentall, R. P., Reid, D., & Faragher, E. B. (1998). A comparison of the long-term effectiveness of distraction and focusing in the treatment of auditory hallucinations. *The British Journal of Medical Psychology, 71 (Pt 3)*, 339–349.

Haddock, G., & Tarrier, N. (1998). Assessment and formulation in the cognitive behavioural treatment of psychosis. In N. Tarrier, A. Wells & G. Haddock (Eds.), *Treating complex cases: The cognitive behavioural approach* (pp. 155–175). Chichester, UK: Wiley.

Hahlweg, K. (2006). *Familienbetreuung schizophrener Patienten*. Goettingen, Germany: Hogrefe.

Hahlweg, K., & Wiedemann, G. (2002). Principles and results of family therapy in schizophrenia. In A. Schaub (Ed.), *New family interventions and associated research in psychiatric disorders* (pp. 155–173). Wien, Austria: Springer Verlag.

Hahlweg K., & Wiedmann G. (1999) Principles and results of family therapy in schizophrenia. *European Archives of Psychiatry and Clinical Neuroscience, 249* (Suppl. 4), 108–115.

Harvey, P. D. (2006). Cognitive and functional effects of atypical antipsychotic medications. *The Journal of Clinical Psychiatry, 67*(10), e13.

Heaton, R., Paulsen, J. S., McAdams, L. A., Kuck, J., Zisook, S., Braff, D., et al. (1994). Neuropsychological deficits in schizophrenics: Relationship to age, chronicity, and dementia. *Archives of General Psychiatry, 51*(6), 469–476.

Heinssen, R. K. (2002). Improving medication compliance of a patient with schizophrenia through collaborative behavioral therapy. *Psychiatric Services, 53*(3), 255–257.

Herrmann-Doig, T., Maude D., & Edwards J. (2003). *Systematic treatment of persistent psychosis (STOPP): A psychological approach of facilitating recovery in young people with first-episode psychosis*. London, UK: Martin Dunitz, Taylor & Francis Group.

Herz, M. I., Lamberti, J. S., Mintz, J., Scott, R., O'Dell, S. P., McCartan, L., et al. (2000). A program for relapse prevention in schizophrenia: a controlled study. *Archives of General Psychiatry, 57*(3), 277–283.

Hodge, M. A., Siciliano, D., Withey, P., Moss, B., Moore, G., Judd, G., et al. (2008). A randomized controlled trial of cognitive remediation in schizophrenia. *Schizophrenia Bulletin, 36*(2), 419–427.

Hofer, A., Rettenbacher, M. A., Edlinger, M., Kemmler, G., Widschwendter, C. G., & Fleischhacker, W. W. (2007). Subjective response and attitudes toward antipsychotic drug therapy during the initial treatment period: a prospective follow-up study in patients with schizophrenia. *Acta Psychiatrica Scandinavia, 116*(5), 354–361.

Hogarty, G. E. (2002). *Personal therapy for schizophrenia and related disorders: A guide to individualized treatment*. New York, NY: Guilford Press.

Hogarty, G. E., Flesher, S., Ulrich, R., Carter, M., Greenwald, D., Pogue-Geile, M., et al. (2004). Cognitive enhancement therapy for schizophrenia: Effects of a 2-year randomized trial on cognition and behavior. *Archives of General Psychiatry, 61*(9), 866–876.

Hogarty, G. E., Goldberg, S. C., & Schooler, N. R. (1974). Drug and sociotherapy in the aftercare of schizophrenic patients III. Adjustment of nonrelapsed patients. *Archives of General Psychiatry, 31*(5), 609–618.

Hogarty, G. E., Kornblith, S. J., Greenwald, D., DiBarry, A. L., Cooley, S., Flesher, S., et al. (1995). Personal therapy: A disorder-relevant psychotherapy for schizophrenia. *Schizophrenia Bulletin, 21*(3), 379–393.

Houthoofd, S. A., Morrens, M., & Sabbe, B. G. (2008). Cognitive and psychomotor effects of risperidone in schizophrenia and schizoaffective disorder. *Clinical Therapeutics, 30*(9), 1565–1589.

Jackson, H. J., McGorry, P. D., Edwards, J., Hulbert, C., Henry, L., Harrigan, S., et al. (2005). A controlled trial of cognitively oriented psychotherapy for early psychosis (COPE) with four-year follow-up readmission data. *Psychological Medicine, 35*(9), 1295–1306.

Jackson, H. J., McGorry, P. D., Henry, L., Edwards, J., Hulbert, C., Harrigan, S., et al. (2001). Cognitively oriented psychotherapy for early psychosis (COPE): A 1-year follow-up. *The British Journal of Clinical Psychology 40*(Pt 1), 57–70.

Jackson, H. J., McGorry, P. D., Killackey, E., Bendall, S., Allott, K., Dudgeon, P., et al. (2008). Acute-phase and 1-year follow-up results of a randomized controlled trial of CBT versus befriending for first-episode psychosis: The ACE project. *Psychological Medicine, 38*(5), 725–735.

Jann, M. W. (2004). Implications for atypical antipsychotics in the treatment of schizophrenia: Neurocognition effects and a neuroprotective hypothesis. *Pharmacotherapy, 24*(12), 1759–1783.

Keefe, R. S., Seidman, L. J., Christensen, B. K., Hamer, R. M., Sharma, T., Sitskoorn, M. M., et al. (2004). Comparative effect of atypical and conventional antipsychotic drugs on neurocognition in first-episode psychosis: A randomized, double-blind trial of olanzapine versus low doses of haloperidol. *The American Journal of Psychiatry, 161*(6), 985–995.

Keefe, R. S., Silva, S. G., Perkins, D. O., & Lieberman, J. A. (1999). The effects of atypical antipsychotic drugs on neurocognitive impairment in schizophrenia: A review and meta-analysis. *Schizophrenia Bulletin, 25*(2), 201–222.

Kemp, R., Hayward, P., Applewhaite, G., Everitt, B., & David, A. (1996). Compliance therapy in psychotic patients: Randomised controlled trial. *British Medical Journal 312*(7027), 345–349.

Kern, R. S., Glynn, S. M., Horan, W. P., & Marder, S. R. (2009). Psychosocial treatments to promote functional recovery in schizophrenia. *Schizophrenia Bulletin, 35*(2), 347–361.

Kern, R. S., Green, M. F., Mintz, J., & Liberman, R. P. (2003). Does ‚errorless learning' compensate for neurocognitive impairments in the work rehabilitation of persons with schizophrenia? *Psychological Medicine, 33*(3), 433–442.

Kern, R. S., Liberman, R. P., Kopelowicz, A., Mintz, J., & Green, M. F. (2002). Applications of errorless learning for improving work performance in persons with schizophrenia. *The American Journal of Psychiatry, 159*(11), 1921–1926.

Kingdon, D. (1998). Cognitive behavioral therapy of psychosis: Complexities in engagement and therapy. In N. Tarrier, A. Wells, & G. Haddock (Eds.), *Treating complex cases: The cognitive behavioural therapy approach* (pp. 176–194). Chichester, UK: Wiley.

Kingdon, D. G., & Turkington, D. (2005). *Cognitive therapy of schizophrenia.* New York, NY: Guilford Press.

Kleim, B., Vauth, R., Stieglitz, R. D., Corrigan, P. W., & Hayward, P. (2007). Perceived stigma predicts low self-efficacy and poor coping in schizophrenia. *Journal of Mental Health, 16,* 1–10

Krabbendam, L., & Aleman, A. (2003). Cognitive rehabilitation in schizophrenia: A quantitative analysis of controlled studies. *Psychopharmacology, 169*(3–4), 376–382.

Kreutz, G., Bongard, S., Rohrmann, S., Hodapp, V., & Grebe, D. (2004). Effects of choir singing or listening on secretory immunoglobulin A, cortisol, and emotional state. *Journal of Behavioral Medicine, 27*(6), 623–635.

Kreyenbuhl, J., Buchanan, R. W., Dickerson, F. B., & Dixon, L. B. (2010). The Schizophrenia Patient Outcomes Research Team (PORT): Updated treatment recommendations 2009. *Schizophrenia Bulletin, 36*(1), 94–103.

Kumari, V., Fannon, D., Ffytche, D. H., Raveendran, V., Antonova, E., Premkumar, P., et al. (2010). Functional MRI of verbal self-monitoring in schizophrenia: performance and illness-specific effects. *Schizophrenia Bulletin, 36*(4), 740–755.

Kumari, V., Peters, E. R., Fannon, D., Antonova, E., Premkumar, P., Anilkumar, A. P., et al. (2009). Dorsolateral prefrontal cortex activity predicts responsiveness to cognitive-behavioral therapy in schizophrenia. *Biological Psychiatry, 66*(6), 594–602.

Kurtz, M. M., Moberg, P. J., Gur, R. C., & Gur, R. E. (2001). Approaches to cognitive remediation of neuropsychological deficits in schizophrenia: A review and meta-analysis. *Neuropsychology Review, 11*(4), 197–210.

Kurtz, M. M., Seltzer, J. C., Fujimoto, M., Shagan, D. S., & Wexler, B. E. (2009). Predictors of change in life skills in schizophrenia after cognitive remediation. *Schizophrenia Research, 107*(2–3), 267–274.

Leucht, S., & Heres, S. (2006). Epidemiology, clinical consequences, and psychosocial treatment of nonadherence in schizophrenia. *Journal Clinical Psychiatry, 67 Suppl 5,* 3–8.

Leventhal, H., & Watts, J. C. (1966). Sources of resistance to fear-arousing communications on smoking and lung cancer. *Journal of Personality and Social Psychology, 34*(2), 155–175.

Lincoln, T. M., Wilhelm, K., & Nestoriuc, Y. (2007). Effectiveness of psychoeducation for relapse, symptoms, knowledge, adherence and functioning in psychotic disorders: A meta-analysis. *Schizophrenia Research, 96*(1–3), 232–245.

Linehan, M. M. (1993). *Skills training manual for treating borderline personality disorder.* New York, NY: Guilford Press.

Little, P., Everitt, H., Williamson, I., Warner, G., Moore, M., Gould, C., et al. (2001). Observational study of effect of patient centredness and positive approach on outcomes of general practice consultations. *British Medical Journal 323*(7318), 908–911.

Liu-Seifert, H., Adams, D. H., Ascher-Svanum, H., Faries, D. E., & Kinon, B. J. (2007). Patient perception of medication benefit and early treatment discontinuation in a 1-year study of patients with schizophrenia. *Patient Preference and Adherence, 1*, 9–17.

Liu-Seifert, H., Adams, D. H., & Kinon, B. J. (2005). Discontinuation of treatment of schizophrenic patients is driven by poor symptom response: A pooled post-hoc analysis of four atypical antipsychotic drugs. *BioMed Central Medicine, 3*, 21.

Lynch, D., Laws, K. R., & McKenna, P. J. (2010). Cognitive behavioural therapy for major psychiatric disorder: does it really work? A meta-analytical review of well-controlled trials. *Psychological Medicine, 40*(1), 9–24.

Malik, N., Kingdon, D., Pelton, J., Mehta, R., & Turkington, D. (2009). Effectiveness of brief cognitive-behavioral therapy for schizophrenia delivered by mental health nurses: Relapse and recovery at 24 months. *The Journal of Clinical Psychiatry, 70*(2), 201–207.

Marshall, M., & Rathbone, J. (2006). Early intervention for psychosis. *Cochrane Database of Systematic Reviews (Online)*(4), CD004718.

McCabe, R., Heath, C., Burns, T., & Priebe, S. (2002). Engagement of patients with psychosis in the consultation: Conversation analytic study. *British Medical Journal 325*(7373), 1148–1151.

McEvoy, J. P., Johnson, J., Perkins, D., Lieberman, J. A., Hamer, R. M., Keefe, R. S., et al. (2006). Insight in first-episode psychosis. *Psychological Medicine, 36*(10), 1385–1393.

McGorry, P. D., Killackey, E., & Yung, A. R. (2007). Early intervention in psychotic disorders: Detection and treatment of the first episode and the critical early stages. *The Medical Journal of Australia, 187*(7 Suppl), S8–S10.

McGorry, P. D., Yung, A. R., Phillips, L. J., Yuen, H. P., Francey, S., Cosgrave, E. M., et al. (2002). Randomized controlled trial of interventions designed to reduce the risk of progression to first-episode psychosis in a clinical sample with subthreshold symptoms. *Archives of General Psychiatry, 59*(10), 921–928.

McGurk, S. R., Mueser, K. T., & Pascaris, A. (2005). Cognitive training and supported employment for persons with severe mental illness: One-year results from a randomized controlled trial. *Schizophrenia Bulletin, 31*(4), 898–909.

McGurk, S. R., Twamley, E. W., Sitzer, D. I., McHugo, G. J., & Mueser, K. T. (2007). A meta-analysis of cognitive remediation in schizophrenia. *The American Journal of Psychiatry, 164*(12), 1791–1802.

Medalia, A., Revheim, N., & Herlands, T. (2009). *Cognitive remediation for psychological disorders, therapist guide.* New York, NY: Oxford University Press.

Meltzer, H. Y., & McGurk, S. R. (1999). The effects of clozapine, risperidone, and olanzapine on cognitive function in schizophrenia. *Schizophrenia Bulletin, 25*(2), 233–255.

Miller, W. R., & Rollnick, S. (2002). *Motivational interviewing: Preparing people for change.* New York, NY: Guilford Press.

Mojtabai, R., Lavelle, J., Gibson, P. J., & Bromet, E. J. (2003). Atypical antipsychotics in first admission schizophrenia: Medication continuation and outcomes. *Schizophrenia Bulletin, 29*(3), 519–530.

Morrison, A. P. (1998). Cognitive behavioral therapy for psychotic symptoms in schizophrenia. In N. Tarrier, A. Wells, & G. Haddock (Eds.), *Treating complex cases: The cognitive behavioural therapy approach* (pp. 195–216). Chichester, UK: Wiley.

Morrison, A. P., & Barratt, S. (2010). What are the components of CBT for psychosis? A Delphi study. *Schizophrenia Bulletin, 36*(1), 136–142.

Morrison, A. P., Bentall, R. P., French, P., Walford, L., Kilcommons, A., Knight, A., et al. (2002). Randomised controlled trial of early detection and cognitive therapy for preventing transition to psychosis in high-risk individuals: Study design and interim analysis of transition rate and psychological risk factors. *The British Journal of Psychiatry Supplement, 43*, s78–s84.

Morrison, A. P., French, P., Walford, L., Lewis, S. W., Kilcommons, A., Green, J., et al. (2004). Cognitive therapy for the prevention of psychosis in people at ultra-high risk: Randomised controlled trial. *185*, 291–297.

Nasar, S. (1998). *A beautiful mind: The Life of mathematical genius and Nobel Laureate John Nash*. US: Touchstone (Simon & Schuster).

National Institute for Health and Clinical Excellence (2009). *Core interventions in the treatment and management of schizophrenia in primary and secondary care (update)*. London, UK: NICE.

Nelson, H. E. (1997). *Cognitive behavioural therapy with schizophrenia: A practical manual*. Cheltenham, UK: Stanley Thrones Ltd.

Palmer, B. W., Heaton, R. K., Paulsen, J. S., Kuck, J., Braff, D., Harris, M. J., et al. (1997). Is it possible to be schizophrenic yet neuropsychologically normal? *Neuropsychology, 11*(3), 437–446.

Penn, D. L., Meyer, P. S., Evans, E., Wirth, R. J., Cai, K., & Burchinal, M. (2009). A randomized controlled trial of group cognitive-behavioral therapy vs. enhanced supportive therapy for auditory hallucinations. *Schizophrenia Research, 109*(1–3), 52–59.

Perkins, D. O., Gu, H., Weiden, P. J., McEvoy, J. P., Hamer, R. M., & Lieberman, J. A. (2008). Predictors of treatment discontinuation and medication nonadherence in patients recovering from a first episode of schizophrenia, schizophreniform disorder, or schizoaffective disorder: A randomized, double-blind, flexible-dose, multicenter study. *The Journal of Clinical Psychiatry, 69*(1), 106–113.

Perkins, D. O., Johnson, J. L., Hamer, R. M., Zipursky, R. B., Keefe, R. S., Centorrhino, F., et al. (2006). Predictors of antipsychotic medication adherence in patients recovering from a first psychotic episode. *Schizophrenia Research, 83*(1), 53–63.

Pitschel-Walz, G., Bauml, J., Bender, W., Engel, R. R., Wagner, M., & Kissling, W. (2006). Psychoeducation and compliance in the treatment of schizophrenia: results of the Munich Psychosis Information Project Study. *Journal Clinical Psychiatry, 67*(3), 443–452.

Premkumar, P., Fannon, D., Kuipers, E., Peters, E. R., Anilkumar, A. P., Simmons, A., et al. (2009). Structural magnetic resonance imaging predictors of responsiveness to cognitive behaviour therapy in psychosis. *Schizophrenia Research, 115*(2–3), 146–155.

Rathod, S., Kingdon, D., Smith, P., & Turkington, D. (2005). Insight into schizophrenia: the effects of cognitive behavioural therapy on the components of insight and association with sociodemographics: Data on a previously published randomised controlled trial. *Schizophrenia Research, 74*(2–3), 211–219.

Rector, N. A., & Beck, A. T. (2002). Cognitive therapy for schizophrenia: From conceptualization to intervention. *Canadian Journal of Psychiatry, 47*, 39–48.

Rettenbacher, M. A., Burns, T., Kemmler, G., & Fleischhacker, W. W. (2004). Schizophrenia: Attitudes of patients and professional carers towards the illness and antipsychotic medication. *Pharmacopsychiatry, 37*(3), 103–109.

Ridgely, M. S., Goldman, H. H., & Willenbring, M. (1990). Barriers to the care of persons with dual diagnoses: organizational and financing issues. *Schizophrenia Bulletin, 16*(1), 123–132.

Romme, M., & Escher, S. (2000). *Making sense of voices: A guide for mental health professionals working with voicehearers*. London, UK: Mind Publications.

Rummel-Kluge, C., & Kissling, W. (2008). Psychoeducation in schizophrenia: new developments and approaches in the field. *Current Opinion in Psychiatry, 21*(2), 168–172.

Rummel-Kluge, C., Pitschel-Walz, G., Bauml, J., & Kissling, W. (2006). Psychoeducation in schizophrenia: Results of a survey of all psychiatric institutions in Germany, Austria, and Switzerland. *Schizophrenia Bulletin, 32*(4), 765–775.

Safran, J. D., & Muran, J. C. (2000). *Negotiating the therapeutic alliance: A relational treatment guide*. New York, NY: Guilford Press.

Sensky, T., Turkington, D., Kingdon, D., Scott, J. L., Scott, J., Siddle, R., et al. (2000). A randomized controlled trial of cognitive-behavioral therapy for persistent symptoms in schizophrenia resistant to medication. *Archives of General Psychiatry, 57*(2), 165–172.

Sharma, S, & Harvey, P. D. (2000). Cognitive enhancement as a treatment strategy in schizophrenia. In S. Sharma & P. D. Harvey (Eds.), *Cognition in schizophrenia: Impairments, importance, and treatment strategies* (pp. 286–302). New York, NY: Oxford University Press.

Solomon P. (2000). Interventions for families of individuals with schizophrenia: maximizing benefits for the relatives. *Disease Management and Health Outcomes, 8*, 211–221.

Spaulding, W. D., Fleming, S. K., Reed, D., Sullivan, M., Storzbach, D., & Lam, M. (1999). Cognitive functioning in schizophrenia: Implications for psychiatric rehabilitation. *Schizophrenia Bulletin, 25*(2), 275–289.

Splitter, C. (2003). Stimmen aus dem Off. Feature am 11.6.2003. Berlin: Deutschlandradio.

Swartz, M. S., Wagner, H. R., Swanson, J. W., Stroup, T. S., McEvoy, J. P., McGee, M., et al. (2006). Substance use and psychosocial functioning in schizophrenia among new enrollees in the NIMH CATIE study. *Psychiatric Services (Washington, D.C), 57*(8), 1110–1116.

Tarrier, N., Beckett, R., Harwood, S., Baker, A., Yusupoff, L., & Ugarteburu, I. (1993). A trial of two cognitive-behavioural methods of treating drug-resistant residual psychotic symptoms in schizophrenic patients: Part I: Outcome. *The British Journal of Psychiatry, 162*, 524–532.

Tarrier, N., Lewis, S., Haddock, G., Bentall, R., Drake, R., Kinderman, P., et al. (2004). Cognitive-behavioural therapy in first-episode and early schizophrenia: 18-month follow-up of a randomised controlled trial. *The British Journal of Psychiatry, 184*, 231–239.

Turkington, D., Kingdon, D., Rathod, S., Hammond, K., Pelton, J., & Mehta, R. (2006a). Outcomes of an effectiveness trial of cognitive-behavioural intervention by mental health nurses in schizophrenia. *The British Journal of Psychiatry, 189*, 36–40.

Turkington, D., Kingdon, D., & Turner, T. (2002). Effectiveness of a brief cognitive-behavioural therapy intervention in the treatment of schizophrenia. *The British Journal of Psychiatry, 180*, 523–527.

Turkington, D., Kingdon, D., & Weiden, P. J. (2006b). Cognitive behavioral therapy for schizophrenia. *The American Journal of Psychiatry, 163*, 365–373.

Twamley, E. W., Jeste, D. V., & Bellack, A. S. (2003). A review of cognitive training in schizophrenia. *Schizophrenia Bulletin, 29*(2), 359–382.

Vauth, R., Corrigan, P. W., Clauss, M., Dietl, M., Dreher-Rudolph, M., Stieglitz, R. D., et al. (2005). Cognitive strategies versus self-management skills as adjunct to vocational rehabilitation. *Schizophrenia Bulletin, 31*(1), 55–66.

Vauth, R., Dietl, M., Stieglitz, R. D., & Olbrich, H. M. (2000). [Cognitive remediation: A new chance in rehabilitation of schizophrenic disorders?] [article in German]. *Der Nervenarzt, 71*(1), 19–29.

Vauth, R., Kleim, B., Wirtz, M., & Corrigan, P. W. (2007). Self-efficacy and empowerment as outcomes of self-stigmatizing and coping in schizophrenia. *Psychiatry Research, 150*(1), 71–80.

Velligan, D. I., Draper, M., Stutes, D., Maples, N., Mintz, J., Tai, S., et al. (2009a). Multimodal cognitive therapy: Combining treatments that bypass cognitive deficits and deal with reasoning and appraisal biases. *Schizophrenia Bulletin, 35*(5), 884–893.

Velligan, D. I., Kern, R. S., & Gold, J. M. (2006a). Cognitive rehabilitation for schizophrenia and the putative role of motivation and expectancies. *Schizophrenia Bulletin, 32*(3), 474–485.

Velligan, D. I., Lam, Y. W., Glahn, D. C., Barrett, J. A., Maples, N. J., Ereshefsky, L., et al. (2006b). Defining and assessing adherence to oral antipsychotics: A review of the literature. *Schizophrenia Bulletin, 32*(4), 724–742.

Velligan, D. I., & Miller, A. L. (1999). Cognitive dysfunction in schizophrenia and its importance to outcome: The place of atypical antipsychotics in treatment. *The Journal of Clinical Psychiatry, 60 Suppl 23*, 25–28.

Velligan, D. I., Mueller, J., Wang, M., Dicocco, M., Diamond, P. M., Maples, N. J., et al. (2006c). Use of environmental supports among patients with schizophrenia. *Psychiatric Services (Washington, D.C), 57*(2), 219–224.

Velligan, D. I., Weiden, P. J., Sajatovic, M., Scott, J., Carpenter, D., Ross, R., et al. (2009b). The expert consensus guideline series: Adherence problems in patients with serious and persistent mental illness. *Journal of Clinical Psychiatry, 70 Suppl 4*, 1–46; quiz 47–48.

Watzlawick, P. (1989). [Is psychotherapy what we call "psychotherapy"?] [article in German]. *Psychotherapie, Psychosomatik, Medizinische Psychologie, 39*(9–10), 323–327.

Weiden, P. J. (2006). Switching in the era of atypical antipsychotics: An updated review. *Postgraduate Medicine,* (Suppl. September), 27-44.

Weiden, P. J. (2007). Understanding and addressing adherence issues in schizophrenia: From theory to practice. *Journal of Clinical Psychiatry, 68 Suppl 14*, 14–19.

Weiden, P. J., Buckley, P. F., & Grody, M. (2007). Understanding and treating „first-episode" schizophrenia. *The Psychiatric Clinics of North America, 30*(3), 481–510.

Weiden, P. J, Burkholder, P, Schooler, NR, Weedon, J, Uzenoff, S, & Turkington, D. (2006b). *Improving antipsychotic adherence in schizophrenia: A randomized pilot study of a brief CBT-based intervention.* Paper presented at the ACNP, Boca Raton, Florida.

Weiden, P. J., Kozma, C., Grogg, A., & Locklear, J. (2004). Partial compliance and risk of rehospitalization among California medicaid patients with schizophrenia. *Psychiatric Services, 55*(8), 886–891.

Weiden, P. J., Preskorn, S. H., Fahnestock, P. A., Carpenter, D., Ross R., & Docherty J. P. (2007). Translating the psychopharmacology of antipsychotics to individualized treatment for severe mental illness: A roadmap. *Journal of Clinical Psychiatry, 68* (Suppl 7), 1–48.

Weiden P. J., Rapkin B., Mott T., Zygmunt A., Goldman D., & Frances A. (1994). Rating of Medication Influences (ROMI) scale in schizophrenia. *Schizophrenia Bulletin, 20,* 297–310.

Weiden, P. J., Schooler, N. R., Goldfinger, S., & al., et. (2006a). Acceptance of maintenance antipsychotic recommendation for patients with "first-episode" schizophrenia: preliminary results from an effectiveness study of oral vs. long-acting atypical antipsychotics. *Psychiatric Services.* New York, US.

Weinberger, D. R., Aloia, M. S., Goldberg, T. E., & Berman, K. F. (1994). The frontal lobes and schizophrenia. *The Journal of Neuropsychiatry and Clinical Neurosciences, 6*(4), 419–427.

Weiss, R. D., Griffin, M. L., Kolodziej, M. E., Greenfield, S. F., Najavits, L. M., Daley, D. C., et al. (2007). A randomized trial of integrated group therapy versus group drug counseling for patients with bipolar disorder and substance dependence. *The American Journal of Psychiatry, 164*(1), 100–107.

Wiedl, K. H. (1999). Rehab rounds: cognitive modifiability as a measure of readiness for rehabilitation. *Psychiatric Services (Washington, D.C.), 50*(11), 1411–1413, 1419.

Woods, S. W., Addington, J., Cadenhead, K. S., Cannon, T. D., Cornblatt, B. A., Heinssen, R., et al. (2009). Validity of the prodromal risk syndrome for first psychosis: findings from the North American Prodrome Longitudinal Study. *Schizophrenia Bulletin, 35*(5), 894–908.

Wykes, T., Hayward, P., Thomas, N., Green, N., Surguladze, S., Fannon, D., et al. (2005). What are the effects of group cognitive behaviour therapy for voices? A randomised control trial. *Schizophrenia Research, 77*(2–3), 201–210.

Wykes, T., Reeder, C., Williams, C., Corner, J., Rice, C., & Everitt, B. (2003). Are the effects of cognitive remediation therapy (CRT) durable? Results from an exploratory trial in schizophrenia. *Schizophrenia Research, 61*(2–3), 163–174.

Wykes, T., Steel, C., Everitt, B., & Tarrier, N. (2008). Cognitive behavior therapy for schizophrenia: Effect sizes, clinical models, and methodological rigor. *Schizophrenia Bulletin, 34*(3), 523–537.

Zimmermann, G., Favrod, J., Trieu, V. H., & Pomini, V. (2005). The effect of cognitive behavioral treatment on the positive symptoms of schizophrenia spectrum disorders: A meta-analysis. *Schizophrenia Research, 77*(1), 1–9.

Appendix

Coping Interview for Voice Hearing*

It is important that you write answers to each of the questions in as much detail as you can. Come back to questions if you are unsure, or if you want to add to them later. This profile of your experiences, we feel should be central to any plan you develop to work with your voices. You need to try ways of recording your experiences. If you have a plan of support with a professional, then this worksheet can help you both to ensure that any support you can get is geared around your way of working.

Your ways of working with voices

What things have you tried that have worked (including help from others)?

____

____

____

Support: What help would you have liked to have been offered?

What, if anything, can professionals offer to you?

____

____

____

How would you like this help? When & Where?

____

____

____

Who should do what?

____

____

____

*Adapted from Coleman, R., & Smith, M. (1997). Accepting and Beginning to Live With Voices. In *Working With Voices Working with voices: Victim to victor* (pp. 37–43). Stockport, UK: Handsell Publishing

What should not happen?

Is there anything that you would not like to happen to you if you are suffering from the effects of the voices?

Understanding voices

If, after the work you have done, you are able to answer the following questions, then it could help you to develop a strategy to understand and work with the voices so that you are able to organize your life with them.

The beginning:
Do you know the reasons for your voices?

The explanation:
Do you know why the voices communicate with you?

The meaning:
Do you know what they mean to you?

Exploring your voices

Throughout the next few pages remember: Think small steps. Don't be too ambitious.

Have you spent time exploring the voices and not just listening to what they say?

Do you know how to work with them for your benefit, to take some control?

Have you explored if any of the voices are related to your life events?

Have you explored ways of dealing with the feelings you experience as a results of these life events?

Have you tried negotiating with the voices? If not, why not?

Are any of your voices reasonable?

Do you have any allies in your voices?

You need to build your strengths from your alliances with the positive aspects of your voices. Are there times when they are reasonable?

____

____

____

Can you refuse to listen to the voices until they are reasonable? Have you tried it?

____

____

____

Structuring time

Have you set time aside to work with the voices?

____

____

____

Have you set time aside to listen to the voices?

____

____

____

Please describe how you have tried and what has been successful when organizing time spent with the voice (s).

____

____

____

Tuning in

Are there positive voices you want to work with?

____

____

____

Positive voices can have positive outcomes. Can you use one voice to help you with the ones that you do not want to listen to?

____

____

____

Can you focus on one voice? Can you be selective?

____

____

____

Can you exclude other voices by focusing on only one?

____

____

____

How do you do this?

____

____

____

Psychotic Symptom Rating Scales (PSYRATS)**

A. Auditory Hallucinations

1. Frequency
0   Voices not present, or present less than once a week
1   Voices occur at least once a week
2   Voices occur at least once a day
3   Voices occur at least once an hour
4   Voices occur continuously or almost continuously, i.e., stop for only a few seconds or minutes

2. Duration
0   Voices not present
1   Voices last for a few seconds, fleeting voices
2   Voices last for several minutes
3   Voices last for at least one hour
4   Voices last for hours at a time

3. Location
0   No voices present
1   Voices sound like they are inside head only
2   Voices outside the head, but close to ears or head. Voices inside the head may also be present
3   Voices sound like they are inside or close to ears and outside head away from ears
4   Voices sound like they are from outside the head only

4. Loudness
0   Voices not present
1   Quieter than own voice, whispers
2   About same loudness as own voice
3   Louder than own voice
4   Extremely loud, shouting

5. Beliefs regarding origin of voices
0   Voices not present
1   Believes voices to be solely internally generated and related to self
2   Holds <50% conviction that voices originate from external causes
3   Holds >50% conviction (but <100%) that voices originate from external causes
4   Believes voices are solely due to external causes (100% conviction)

6. Amount of negative content of voices
0   No unpleasant content
1   Occasional unpleasant content (<10%)
2   Minority of voice content is unpleasant or negative (<50%)
3   Majority of voice content is unpleasant or negative (>50%)
4   All of voice content is unpleasant or negative

** Haddock, G., McCarron, J., Tarrier, N., & Faragher, E. B. (1999). Scales to Measure Dimensions of Hallucinations and Delusions: The Psychotic Symptom Rating Scales (PSYRATS). *Psychological Medicine, 29,* 879–889.

7. Degree of negative content

0   Not unpleasant or negative
1   Some degree of negative content, but not personal comments relating to self or family – e.g., swear words or comments not directed to self, e.g., "the milkman's ugly"
2   Personal verbal abuse, comments on behavior, e.g., "shouldn't do that or say that"
3   Personal verbal abuse relating to self-concept, e.g., "you're lazy, ugly, mad, perverted"
4   Personal threats to self, e.g., threats to harm self or family, extreme instructions or commands to harm self or others

8. Amount of distress

0   Voices not distressing at all
1   Voices occasionally distressing, majority not distressing (<10%)
2   Minority of voices distressing (<50%)
3   Majority of voices distressing, minority not distressing (>50%)
4   Voices always distressing

9. Intensity of distress

0   Voices not distressing at all
1   Voices slightly distressing
2   Voices are distressing to a moderate degree
3   Voices are very distressing, although subject could feel worse
4   Voices are extremely distressing, feel the worst he/she could possibly feel

10. Disruption to life caused by voices

0   No disruption to life, able to maintain social and family relationships (if present).
1   Voices cause minimal amount of disruption to life, e.g., interfere with concentration although able to maintain daytime activity and social and family relationships and be able to maintain independent living without support.
2   Voices cause moderate amount of disruption to life causing some disturbance to daytime activity and/or family or social activities. The patient is not in hospital although may live in supported accommodation or receive additional help with daily living skills.
3   Voices cause severe disruption to life so that hospitalization is usually necessary. The patient is able to maintain some daily activities, self-care, and relationships while in hospital. The patient may also be in supported accommodation but experiencing severe disruption of life in terms of activities, daily living skills, and/or relationships.
4   Voices cause complete disruption of daily life requiring hospitalization. The patient is unable to maintain any daily activities and social relationships. Self-care is also severely disrupted.

11. Controllability of voices

0   Subject believes they can have control over the voices and can always bring on or dismiss them at will
1   Subject believes they can have some control over the voices on the majority of occasions
2   Subject believes they can have some control over their voices approximately half of the time
3   Subject believes they can have some control over their voices but only occasionally. The majority of the time the subject experiences voices that are uncontrollable
4   Subject has no control over when the voices occur and cannot dismiss or bring them on at all

B Delusions

1. Amount of preoccupation with delusions
0   No delusions, or delusions which the subject thinks about less than once a week
1   Subject thinks about beliefs at least once a week
2   Subject thinks about beliefs at least once a day
3   Subject thinks about beliefs at least once an hour
4   Subject thinks about delusions continuously or almost continuously

2. Duration of preoccupation with delusions
0   No delusions
1   Thoughts about beliefs last for a few seconds, fleeting thoughts
2   Thoughts about delusions last for several minutes
3   Thoughts about delusions last for at least 1 hour
4   Thoughts about delusions usually last for hours at a time

3. Conviction
0   No conviction at all
1   Very little conviction in reality of beliefs, <10%
2   Some doubts relating to conviction in beliefs, between 10% and 49%
3   Conviction in belief is very strong, between 50% and 99%
4   Conviction is 100%

4. Amount of distress
0   Beliefs never cause distress
1   Beliefs cause distress on the minority of occasions
2   Beliefs cause distress on <50% of occasions
3   Beliefs cause distress on the majority of occasions when they occur between 50% and 99% of time
4   Beliefs always cause distress when they occur

5. Intensity of distress
0   No distress
1   Beliefs cause slight distress
2   Beliefs cause moderate distress
3   Beliefs cause marked distress
4   Beliefs cause extreme distress, could not be worse

6. Disruption to life caused by beliefs
0   No disruption to life, able to maintain independent living with no problems in daily living skills. Able to maintain social and family relationships (if present)
1   Beliefs cause minimal amount of disruption to life, e.g., interferes with concentration although able to maintain daytime activity and social and family relationships and able to maintain independent living without support
2   Beliefs cause moderate amount of disruption to life causing some disturbance to daytime activity and/or family or social activities. The patient is not in hospital although may live in supported accommodation or receive additional help with daily living skills
3   Beliefs cause severe disruption to life so that hospitalization is usually necessary. The patient is able to maintain some daily activities, self-care, and relationships while in hospital. The patient may be also be in supported accommodation but experiencing severe disruption of life in terms of activities, daily living skills, and/or relationships
4   Beliefs cause complete disruption of daily life requiring hospitalization. The patient is unable to maintain any daily activities and social relationships. Self-care is also severely disrupted

BAVQ-R*

There are many people who hear voices. It would help us to find out how you are feeling about your voices by completing this questionnaire. Please read each statement and tick the box which best describes the way you have been feeling in the *past week*.

If you hear more than one voice, please complete the form for the voice that is dominant.

Thank you for your help.

Name: _______________________________

Age: _______________________________

		Disagree	Unsure	Slightly Agree	Strongly Agree
1	My voice is punishing me for something I have done.	❏	❏	❏	❏
2	My voice wants to help me.	❏	❏	❏	❏
3	My voice is very powerful.	❏	❏	❏	❏
4	My voice is persecuting me for no good reason.	❏	❏	❏	❏
5	My voice wants to protect me.	❏	❏	❏	❏
6	My voice seems to know everything about me.	❏	❏	❏	❏
7	My voice is evil.	❏	❏	❏	❏
8	My voice is helping to keep me sane.	❏	❏	❏	❏
9	My voice makes me do things I really don't want to do.	❏	❏	❏	❏
10	My voice wants to harm me.	❏	❏	❏	❏
11	My voice is helping me to develop my special powers or abilities.	❏	❏	❏	❏
12	I cannot control my voices.	❏	❏	❏	❏
13	My voice wants me to do bad things.	❏	❏	❏	❏
14	My voice is helping me to achieve my goal in life.	❏	❏	❏	❏
15	My voice will harm or kill me if I disobey or resist it.	❏	❏	❏	❏
16	My voice is trying to corrupt or destroy me.	❏	❏	❏	❏
17	I am grateful for my voice.	❏	❏	❏	❏
18	My voice rules my life.	❏	❏	❏	❏
19	My voice reassures me.	❏	❏	❏	❏
20	My voice frightens me.	❏	❏	❏	❏
21	My voice makes me happy.	❏	❏	❏	❏
22	My voice makes me feel down.	❏	❏	❏	❏
23	My voice makes me feel angry.	❏	❏	❏	❏
24	My voice makes me feel calm.	❏	❏	❏	❏
25	My voice makes me feel anxious.	❏	❏	❏	❏
26	My voice makes me feel confident.	❏	❏	❏	❏

* Chadwick P., & Taylor, G. (2000). Are deluded people usually prone to illusory correlation? *Behavior Modification, 24*(1), 130–141.

When I hear my voice, <u>usually</u> ...

		Disagree	Unsure	Slightly Agree	Strongly Agree
27	I tell it to leave me alone.	❏	❏	❏	❏
28	I try and take my mind off it.	❏	❏	❏	❏
29	I try and stop it.	❏	❏	❏	❏
30	I do things to prevent it talking.	❏	❏	❏	❏
31	I am reluctant to obey it.	❏	❏	❏	❏
32	I listen to it because I want to.	❏	❏	❏	❏
33	I willingly follow what my voice tells me to do.	❏	❏	❏	❏
34	I have done things to start to get in contact with my voice.	❏	❏	❏	❏
35	I seek the advice of my voice.	❏	❏	❏	❏

Adherence Attitude Interview Worksheet

Suggested Interview Items for Adherence Attitudes
Influence of specific item is scored of 0 = not a factor, 1 = present but minimal influence on (non)adherence; 2 = some influence on (non)adherence, and 3 = strong influence on (non)adherence.

Advantages	Adherence Influence	Disadvantages	Nonadherence Influence
Believes there is an illness that needs to be treated with medication		Does not agree that there is an illness in need of medication	
Taking medication achieves some day-to-day benefits		No noticeable day-to-day benefits associated with taking medication	
Taking medications helps reduce certain distressing symptoms		Continued distress from symptoms despite medication	
Symptoms improved by medication		Attributes symptoms to medication	
Medications help maintaining stability or preventing relapse		Does not believe that there will be a relapse, or does not think stopping medication increases risk of relapse	
Medications help with being more "normal"		Medication interferes with being "normal"	
Side effects are better than other medications previously prescribed		Side effects worse than before, or interfere with functioning	
Medications help facilitate relationships with others		Side effects are visible to others, or interfere with relationships	
Medication has fewer side effects / patient does not feel "medicated"		Distress over a side effect Fear of a future side effect	
Medication helps with achieving life goal(s)		Medication interferes with achieving life goal(s)	
Patient is influenced by family/friend to stay with medication		Patient is influenced by family/friend to go off medication	
Relationship with clinician influences patient to stay adherent		Does not believe in clinician's opinion because of distrust or other relationship problems	
Patient is not concerned about stigma of medication		Patient feels stigmatized by medication	
Feels that staying on medication is useful during episodes of drug/substance use		Patient is using other drugs or alcohol, stops medication during times of use	
Other adherence attitude issues elicited:			

The interview goal is to better understand the person's range of attitudes and motivations concerning medication adherence. **It is not meant to estimate actual adherence behavior. It is not meant to be an adherence intervention at the time the interview is conducted.**

Please be aware of your tone and demeanor when you ask about reasons for adherence and nonadherence. Be curious. Avoid being judgmental. Make sure you cover reasons for adherence as well as reasons for nonadherence. Expect inconsistencies, because many patients have ambivalent beliefs and attitudes, or their attitudes may fluctuate from one day to the next. Focus on understanding attitudes. Try to *avoid making any "corrective" statements during the interview.*

The A-Z of Coping with Voices*

Accept the reality of your voices

Break through the victim barrier

Consider all your options

Develop coping strategies that suit you

Enter into dialogue with your voices

Focus in on your voices

Go to a self-help group

Help others by sharing your experience

Identify the areas in your life that you need to work on

Join activities outside of mental health organizations

Keep a diary

Live your life not your label

Make space for yourself

Negotiate with your voices

Own your voices

Perseverance is the name of the game

Question your voices

Reward yourself when you succeed

Small is beautiful

Take your time – haste can mean failure

Use services to your advantage

Victories have to be fought for

Work on your weaknesses

Xperiment with different coping strategies

You make your decisions, not your voices

Zap your negative voices by gaining control over them

*Adapted from Coleman, R., & Smith, M. (1997). Accepting and Beginning to Live With Voices. In *Working With Voices Working with voices: Victim to victor* (pp. 37–43). Stockport, UK: Handsell Publishing